Comments on
A Headache i

"This is the book to read before you contemplate surgery, drugs or resign yourself to continue to suffer with chronic pelvic pain."

Erik Peper, Ph.D.
Professor and Director
Institute for Holistic Healing Studies
California State University, San Francisco
Past President, Biofeedback Society of America
Author of Make Health Happen

"*A Headache in the Pelvis* is a lamp in the dark human suffering of chronic pelvic pain. This book is a precious document that will help many people."

Robert Blum, M.D.
Director, North Bay Pain Center
Former Chief, Department of Neurosurgery
Marin General Hospital
Marin County, California

"Many pelvic pain patients go from doctor to doctor, specialist to specialist without improvement, often feeling abandoned. A majority of patients with chronic pelvic pain do not respond to conventional therapies (antibiotics and anti-inflammatory drugs) leaving a huge void. Drs. Wise and Anderson offer a therapeutic option that can bring relief to many."

Bart Gershbein, M.D.
Clinical Instructor
Department of Urology
University of California School of Medicine
San Francisco, California

"*A Headache in the Pelvis* is a very important contribution to understanding and treating pelvic pain. It is also an illuminating discussion of the relationship of mental and physical interaction in the production of disease, and an approach to a truly comprehensive treatment of illness that has relevance to a whole range of contemporary morbidities."

Donald L. Fink, M.D.
Professor Emeritus
University of California, San Francisco
School of Medicine

"The work described here by Drs. Wise and Anderson is at the forefront of the understanding and treatment of chronic pelvic pain syndromes like prostatitis. Their approach sees the big picture of these disorders and breaks new ground in our understanding of the subtlety of the mind-body continuum."

A.S. Hadland, M.D.
Director Integrative Medicine
Pain Management Service
Kaiser Permanente

"*A Headache in the Pelvis* is a book which casts an entirely new light upon the serious problem of chronic pelvic pain, and introduces a treatment that offers hope and relief to the many who suffer from it. It is surely "must read" for all who must deal with this debilitating problem as well as all who attempt to treat it."

Martin F. Schwartz, Ph.D.
Research Associate Professor
Department of Surgery
NYU School of Medicine

"This compelling understanding of chronic pelvic pain syndromes offers a new and pioneering approach to its alleviation."

Frank Werblin, Ph.D.
Professor of Neuroscience
University of California, Berkeley

"It is important for the patient to learn all he can about his disease especially if he has prostatitis/chronic pelvic pain syndrome. That is difficult because doctors seldom agree on the cause, cure or treatment. The information contained in *A Headache in the Pelvis* will be essential for these patients."

Mike Hennenfent
President of The Prostatitis Foundation

"This book is something different something not seen before in the field of prostatitis/chronic pelvic pain. This book will take you to a place you have never been before within prostatitis/chronic pelvic pain syndrome. The relaxation techniques, exercise, and myofascial/trigger point release all are outlined and explained in great detail. Examples used to explain various points are truly excellent and enlightening. Pick up this book and you will be taken into a world of relaxation calm and above all a way to possibly ease your symptoms. The authors have created a new portal into the condition and offer you through the book just what they do to help sufferers get better. Lay back relax and you will not be able to put this book down. To suddenly be aware of your pelvic pain in the ways outlined in this book is a truly enlightening experience. This time last year we could not have dreamed it possible to see a book like this on the book shelf.

One of the authors of this book tells you about his own 22 year struggle (which he won) with chronic pelvic pain syndrome (*A Headache in the Pelvis*) so it's from a sufferers perspective at times you will often say to yourself YES I feel like that when reading this book and smile simply because you will feel one thing; the authors understand my problem. Every UK urologist should read this book. If you can afford it you may wish to buy your Doctor a copy."

The British Prostatitis Support Association

"I suffered from prostatitis/chronic pelvic pain syndrome for 3 years and my life became absolutely miserable. I received 4 different diagnoses from 4 urologists, tried over 20 prescription medications, vitamins, and herbs, and underwent several very uncomfortable and expensive procedures, all of which did hardly anything to help my symptoms which had slowly been increasing in intensity over time (sound familiar?) Eventually I met one of the authors of this book, David Wise, and he taught me the techniques described in the book. Slowly I began to heal myself, without any medication. Six months later my symptoms were diminished significantly and nine months later I felt I was healed. It is now 2-1/2 years after I first started to practice these methods and I feel that I have been freed of this horrific condition.

I cannot recommend this book highly enough for those who are still suffering. There are many schools of thought regarding this syndrome and I studied all of them obsessively at one time. I feel very strongly however that over the coming years the ideas in this book will eclipse the other models of this disease and come to be recognized as the most powerful methods for dealing with it as more and more people are seen to have solid and long-lasting benefits. Mine is not the last testimonial you will see. I should say however that it is not a simple or quick solution and it requires a lot of devotion, but chances are the end-result will be your freedom. Best of luck, do not abandon hope until you have given these methods your most sincere effort."

Reader review on Amazon

A Headache in the Pelvis:

A new understanding and treatment

for prostatitis and chronic pelvic pain syndromes

David Wise, Ph.D.   Rodney U. Anderson, M.D.

A Headache in the Pelvis:

*A New Understanding and Treatment
for Prostatitis and Chronic Pelvic Pain Syndromes*

© 2003 David Wise, Ph.D. and Rodney U. Anderson, M.D.

National Center for Pelvic Pain Research
P.O. Box 54
Occidental, CA 95465
Toll Free 866-874-2225
Fax. 707-874-2335

Cover design by
Bob Lee Hickson

Publisher's Cataloging-in-Publication Data
Wise, David Thomas, 1945-
   A headache in the pelvis: a new understanding and treatment of prostatitis and chronic pelvic pain syndromes / David Wise, Rodney U. Anderson. — 3rd ed. — Occidental, CA: National Center for Pelvic Pain Research, 2004, c2003.
   p.; cm.
   ISBN: 0-9727755-2-8
   1. Pelvic pain. 2. Pelvic pain—Treatment. 3. Pelvis—Diseases. 4. Prostatitis—Treatment. I. Anderson, Rodney U. II. Title.
   RC946 .W55 2004
   617.5/5—dc22 0412   2002156599

2 4 6 8 9 7 5 3 1

Third edition

Dedication

This book is dedicated to the many brave men and women who suffer daily from chronic pelvic pain and dysfunction. We hope they will derive benefit from our work.

Summary of Our Understanding

We have identified a group of chronic pelvic pain syndromes that we believe is caused by the overuse of the human instinct to protect the genitals, rectum, and contents of the pelvis from injury or pain by contracting the pelvic muscles. This tendency becomes exaggerated in predisposed individuals and over time results in chronic pelvic pain and dysfunction. The state of chronic constriction creates pain-referring trigger points, reduced blood flow, and an inhospitable environment for the nerves, blood vessels, and structures throughout the pelvic basin. This results in a cycle of tension, anxiety, and pain, which has previously been unrecognized and untreated.

Understanding this tension, anxiety, and pain cycle has allowed us to create an effective treatment. Our program breaks the cycle by rehabilitating the shortened pelvic muscles and connective tissue supporting the pelvic organs while simultaneously using a specific methodology to modify the tendency to tighten the muscles of the pelvic floor under stress.

Table of Contents

Preface to the First Edition

As someone who suffered for twenty-two years with pelvic pain and dysfunction, I conducted a very long and personal research into the subject of this book. Today, I am grateful to have been symptom-free for years.

During the first several years of no pain, I was reluctant to be very public about it. This reluctance was born out of some kind of superstition in me that if I told my story, somehow the blessing of having no more pain would be taken away. I was also hesitant to share the very personal information related to my pelvic pain in a public forum.

Over the years, as I treated others with pelvic pain at Stanford and watched many of them improve, the kind of real improvement like my own that I rarely saw with any other treatment, I became more confident that the method that I used for my own recovery was substantial and should be communicated to people who were suffering as I had. My desire to help those with nowhere to turn, who were suffering as I had, overcame my embarrassment about sharing things most people don't share with others.

I joined with Dr. Rodney Anderson, the renowned neurourologist at Stanford University Medical School, who has been the court of last resort for many people with pelvic pain. Dr. Anderson and I have worked together for eight years in developing the protocol I brought to Stanford. This book is the result of our collaboration.

When I see patients who describe the misery that they are in because they are hurting constantly, I understand. For years, I hurt constantly. More times than I can remember I would wake up in the middle of the night weeping because my pain was so great and I saw no solution for it.

The doctors whom I saw were in the dark about my condition and no one that I knew, except one friend with whom I lost touch, had any idea of what I was going through. There was no internet at that time, no support groups, and little access to any information on my condition. I would go to the medical library at a local hospital, or the medical library at the University of California Medical Center, and pore over old medical journals looking for some kind of clue that might help me. Then, through some serendipity, I found something that worked. Below I share with the reader a little bit of my journey.

When I was 28 years old, I remember sitting in my new office and feeling an uncomfortable sensation in my rectum. The feeling was as if a golf ball was lodged up inside and I could not get it out. No matter how I moved, what exercise I did or diet I tried, this feeling persisted. Along with rectal pain, I found the need to urinate frequently. To my dismay, my bladder never felt quite empty after urination. Intercourse sometimes was uncomfortable and often seemed to exacerbate my symptoms.

I went to see an urologist who gave me both good and bad news. The good news was that he couldn't find anything wrong. There was no infection, no growth or abnormality in the prostate or surrounding area. The bad news was that he couldn't find anything wrong and therefore couldn't help me. He called what I had "prostatosis," which meant, I believed at the time, the discomfort and urinary frequency and urgency that I felt somehow came from the prostate gland, but the prostate gland was normal.

I was lucky to find a kindly doctor. I say I was lucky after seeing many patients, some of whom saw doctors who did invasive procedures, surgeries and put them on courses of antibiotics and medications for years that didn't help. The doctor whom I found was wise enough to recognize that he didn't know what was going on with me and didn't offer any heroic measures despite my suffering.

I would see this doctor regularly, sometimes every three or six months. He would do a prostate exam, extract prostatic fluid, go into another room where he looked at the fluid under a microscope, and then come back into the little examining room I was in and say "It is clear–no infection." I would ask him "Is there anything new being tried, any new research?" He would reply: "No, not now, but I think this gets better as you get older and there is less sexual activity."

His comments were reassuring to me, especially the comment that I would get better. He was however incorrect in telling me that the condition gets better with age, even though I still appreciate this inaccurate statement. I noticed that the more anxious I was, the worse my symptoms got. Being someone who tends toward anxiety, I think I would have had a more difficult time without this doctor's kindly but inaccurate assurance.

I tried everything. I started out with the regular medical treatments of antibiotics, which did not help me. I experimented with diet, cutting out alcohol, coffee and spicy foods on the advice of the physician I was seeing. There was no benefit. Someone told me that certain reflexology pressure points near the ankle could help. I pressed those pressure points to the point of great pain for many months hoping for some relief. I read somewhere that zinc deficiency could cause my problem, and so I took zinc supplements regularly. I tried many sessions of acupuncture, psychotherapy, guided imagery visualization, cutting out alcohol, caffeine and spicy foods, hands on healing and prayer. All made no difference to my condition.

There were some things that helped a little and then stopped helping. Warm baths sometimes took the edge off of my pain. Occasionally, prostate massage temporarily reduced the symptoms but only for a few hours. Eventually when I would return to the doctor, prostate massage failed to have any effect.

The truth is, as I look at it now, nothing really helped in any lasting way. While there was almost always an underlying sense of discomfort, when flare-ups would occur, often after sex, they would last for months and months. Many patients have asked me how I lived with these symptoms for twenty-two years. As I reflect now, there was no magic to it. When times were bad, I muddled through. The cost to my quality of life was very high. When my symptoms were bad, I found myself distracted and I withdrew inwardly from social situations and my loved ones. Miraculously, I never took off work, even though I very much understand how someone would. In the language of current day America, "You do what you gotta do."

My symptoms waxed and waned, though never really went away. After years of having symptoms, I found myself in the fortunate position of not having to work. I had dreamed about this for many years and somehow it became a reality.

The effect of my newfound freedom on my pelvic pain was not what I expected. It never occurred to me that my anxiety would increase. In fact, my symptoms got much worse. More than that, their severity became constant and I found no relief day or night. I well remember lying in bed during a heavy rain storm. Being in a warm bed and hearing the rain on the roof had been one of my pleasures, but during this time there was no pleasure because I could find no escape from the constant aching that I felt.

In my desperation, I began making phone calls to doctors and researchers around the world whose names I took from the medical literature. It was from this desperate search that I discovered a way to eventually stop my symptoms.

After several months of using the protocol described in this book, I occasionally did not feel the need to go to the bathroom for four or five hours. This felt amazing to me. As time went on, I would notice that I was pain-free for brief periods. These periods gradually increased. Later, weeks passed when I had no symptoms.

To my dismay, there were still many flare-ups and my symptoms would return full-blown. The flare-ups, however, lasted a fraction of the time than they used to. I was getting better. Imperceptibly, my regular state became one of no pelvic pain or dysfunction.

I felt normal. I was grateful beyond words for the feeling that everything inside was working right. The joy of feeling normal in my bladder was beyond my ability to communicate. Feeling normal is a peculiar way to describe how I felt because it really doesn't communicate the ease and pleasure I felt about something that most people never even notice and simply take for granted. And aside from close friends being happy that I was feeling good, my sense was that no one really understood how it felt inside me to simply feel normal.

It took over two years for all of the symptoms to go away. To this day, I continue to use the relaxation protocol and I believe it has been essential in my remaining well.

We hope this book brings some clarity and direction to many who suffer from pelvic pain. It is written for those who have no familiarity with medical terminology or research and we include neither footnotes nor a bibliography, although we include a simplified review of literature in Chapter 6.

David Wise, Ph.D.
Sebastopol, California

* * * * *

Many years ago I had the privilege and pleasure of being mentored by one of the giants of American Urology. Dr. Thomas A. Stamey, Chairman of the Department of Urology at Stanford University, introduced me as a resident in training to the problems that men endured with chronic prostatitis. More importantly, he introduced me to a way of evaluating patients with meticulous detail, being curious and mindful of every nuance of symptom and finding. He reiterated continuously the importance of paying attention to detail and being a "thinking" urologist as opposed to mindlessly throwing pills at or cutting your way through a problem. He also showed me through his clinical research methods that it was much better to study a few patients thoroughly than a lot of patients superficially.

Dr. Stamey taught me to look through the microscope and see what human inflammatory cells looked like in the prostatic fluid of men suffering with prostatitis. He got quite excited to demonstrate fat-laden macrophages that exhibited a Maltese-cross appearance under polarized light. He showed me how to carefully segregate the urine specimens from the prostatic fluid to prove whether a patient had true bacterial colonization of the prostate or some contaminant. His seminal publication with our other colleague, Dr. Edwin Meares, still stands as the pivotal work to define prostatic infection.

Unfortunately, no matter how much we have studied this problem of chronic prostatitis and chronic pelvic pain syndrome, in both men and women, three decades later we still do not understand why it happens and how to prevent it. Fortunately my partner Dr. David Wise, a perceptive psychologist, came along and described his experience and discoveries in abating his symptoms after having dealt with his condition for many years. Since that time I have been impressed that this approach helps many more people than pharmaceutical agents or surgery.

This small book is our attempt to convey to the patients suffering from chronic pelvic pain syndromes our genuine concern for their well-being and to describe our experience with an alternative approach to improve or resolve their symptoms. At the same time we attempt to help clarify and explain the controversies and medical investigations ongoing to elucidate the biologic basis of these complaints.

Rodney U. Anderson, M.D., FACS
Stanford, California

Preface to the Second Edition

In a little more than half a year we have sold out of the first hardbound edition of our book. The response to our book has been well beyond our expectations. Our book has been ordered from almost every state in the Union and many countries on every continent in the world. The emails we have gotten have brought home how the problem we describe is not limited to national boundary, culture, or race. The people who suffer from chronic pelvic pain syndromes all undergo the same kinds of symptoms and suffer the same kinds of pain, dysfunction, and anguish.

Most of the letters we have received express their appreciation for having received a new way of understanding and treating certain kinds of chronic pelvic pain. Indeed readers often report that their symptoms tend to reduce after simply reading our book. This may be because the simple reassurance that what they have is not life-threatening can frequently lead to alleviation of symptoms on a short-term basis.

In this new edition, we have included a number of additions. We have updated our research review with the latest important research findings. We have added a chapter that includes a number of reports from patients who have undergone our treatment and who continue to practice our protocol. We have added more stretches that have proven useful. We have included a section describing Respiratory Sinus Arrhythmia breathing that is used preliminary to Paradoxical Relaxation. Importantly, we have published this edition as a paperback for a significantly lower cost.

David Wise, Ph.D.
Rodney U. Anderson, M.D., FACS
September 23, 2003

Preface to the Third Edition

Our book continues to be received with great enthusiasm by many who suffer from chronic pelvic pain. We continue to receive correspondence from people in many different countries who express their gratitude at the possibilities that our book opens up.

This third edition is a significant edition because we have included an extensive written and graphic presentation of our physical therapy protocol. We have updated the section on research to include the latest studies on pelvic pain. We have included a section about what we believe are the common origins of chronic pelvic pain and other disorders including hemorrhoids, anal fissures and constipation, and the possible use of the Stanford protocol for these difficulties. A more extensive discussion of biofeedback is also included as well as an expanded explanation of the technique of *Paradoxical Relaxation.*

During the time of our second edition, we began offering treatment for pelvic pain in the form of a 6-day, 30 hour intensive clinic in which both *Paradoxical Relaxation* and physical therapy are offered on site in California. This format has proved to be the most effective one we have used. We have also begun a new website, www.pelvicpainhelp.com which contains much information about different aspects of our work. We are more enthusiastic about our work than we ever have been in the past and there is slow but growing interest on the part of the medical community.

We have recently submitted an analysis of our experience and outcomes in over 100 men who have used our protocol to a medical journal. Because of the policies of the journal we are not at liberty to publish that information at this time, but we are very pleased with the results and look forward to releasing that information soon.

David Wise, Ph.D.
Rodney U. Anderson, M.D., FACS

Acknowledgements

We wish to acknowledge the inspiration of Dr. Thomas A. Stamey, mentor and teacher at Stanford University, in the Department of Urology, without whose pioneering research into prostatitis, this book would not have been possible.

We also wish to express our gratitude to the following individuals who have helped us in the writing of this book:

Elaine Orenberg Anderson, Harold Wise, Erik Peper, Ruth Dreier, Tiaga Liner, Martin Schwartz, Judith Schwartz, Frank Werblin, Jeanette Potts, Marilyn Freedman, Amanita Rosenbush, Dan Poynter, Suzanne Pregerson, Susan Page, Steve Hadland, Anneke Vanderveen, Walter Blum, Ramana Maharshi, Rhonda Kotarinos, Jean Klein, Michael Aronowitz, Jane Kramer, Mitch Feldman, Kathy Harris, Rick Harvey, Allaudin Mathieu, Larry Rabon, Nathan Segal, Joseph Segal, Clair Sutton, Lindy Woodard, Vivian Aronowitz, Jack Gabriel, Bart Gershbein, June Wise, Shera Wise Silver, Ted Silver, Fay Nathanson, Larry Nathanson, Brian Nathanson, Richard Gevirtz, Byron Katie, Mary Kenney, Harry Kenney, Clair Kenney, Elizabeth Kenney, Steve Wall, Jerome Weiss, Carol Davis, Laura Frazier, Donald Fink, Daniel Fink, Mortecai Mitnik, Judith Klinman, Zepporah Glass, Cinnamon Wise, Helen Wise, Symon Wise, Ron Reneau, Sophia Savalas, Francine Shapiro, Frederick Perls, Jim Simkin, Alan Leveton, Ann Armstrong, Ann Dreyfuss, Leo Zeff, Walter Kaufmann, Milton Rosenberg, Edmund Jacobson, Helene Morcos, Richard Miller, Ann Miller, Larry Bloomberg, Ed Sampson, Phil Curcuruto, Howard Glazer, Nadia Nurhussein, Ellen Vandenberg, Judith Goleman, Rick Larue, Dawn Larue, Donna Spitzer, Rachel Ruch, Daniel Goleman, Diana Schlaufler, Patricia Speier, Marlene Cohen, Susan Todd, Cheri Quincy, Joel Alter, Alan Dreyfuss, Alex Kritz, John Adair, Larry Todd, Stephanie Rosencrans, Cynthia Frank and Sara Seibet-Sawyer. We express our deep appreciation for the seminal work of Dr. Edmund Jacobson for his pioneering work in *Progressive Relaxation* and to Drs. Janet Travell and David Simons for their pioneering work of myofascial/trigger point treatment. We are particularly indebted to Tim Sawyer, P.T., for his great skill and talent in Myofascial/Trigger Point Release of the pelvic floor, who has been our senior consultant in physical therapy in our work at Stanford.

CHAPTER 1

DEFINITIONS AND CATEGORIES

Millions of men and women suffer from pelvic pain, discomfort, or dysfunction. These disorders, which can be called chronic pelvic pain syndromes (CPPS) sometimes, include *rectal, genital, or abdominal pain. These kinds of conditions can also include urinary frequency and urgency as well as discomfort during and after sexual activity.* Historically, these conditions have been given many different names. As a result, they have been thought to have numerous causes.

In the majority of cases, doctors can find little or no physical basis for the symptoms. In this book, we will demonstrate that there may be a simple physical basis for the symptoms and that the seemingly wide array and variability of the symptoms are simply regional expressions of the variety of ways in which the body can react. A treatment protocol has been developed. We no longer treat the symptoms; instead we treat what triggers those symptoms. Our approach substantially reduces or abates symptoms in the majority of patients who undertake our full protocol.

In this book we will use the terms, *a headache in the pelvis, chronic pelvic pain syndrome(s), chronic pelvic pain, pelvic pain*, and *CPPS* synonymously to refer to all the conditions discussed.

Traditional names

In Men

- Prostatitis (National Institutes of Health categories)
  - I   Acute bacterial prostatitis
  - II   Chronic bacterial prostatitis
  - IIIA CPPS nonbacterial inflammatory prostatitis
  - IIIB CPPS nonbacterial non-inflammatory prostatitis
  - IV   Asymptomatic inflammatory prostatitis
- Isolated orchalgia
- Proctalgia fugax

In Women

- Vulvodynia (vulvar vestibulitis)
- Urethral syndrome

In Both Men and Women

- Interstitial cystitis
- Levator ani syndrome
- Pudendal nerve entrapment syndrome

What is common in the different names

The central notion in this book is that there is a *common factor that unites the different names: that there is a common effective treatment for many of them; and that the body and the mind are both involved in the cause and the treatment.*

For many years, chronic pelvic pain syndromes have posed an enigma to the medical community. Nonbacterial prostatitis, for example, has routinely been confused with acute or chronic bacterial prostatitis even though a correct method for diagnosis has been available for years. At the same time, nonbacterial prostatitis tends to be regarded by doctors as a kind of wastebasket category of *functional somatic disorders.* Gross pathology, as measured by the latest medical instruments, has not been able to explain the degree of suffering caused by these disorders. Functional somatic disorders, as we will discuss, implies that the problem lies not in pathology of structure but in a dysfunction of a structure.

What we are proposing in this book is that these conditions are rather like a headache, except the location of the headache is in the pelvis. Hence, *A Headache in the Pelvis* is our title. A further implication from the title is that these disorders are problems of chronic muscle tension, which is often the basis of many headaches. If chronic pelvic pain syndromes are, in fact, a headache in the pelvis, then treatment needs to be radically different from what has traditionally been followed.

A "headache in the pelvis" is the name we are giving to chronic pelvic pain syndromes where no clear pathology has been found. These syndromes often include pain and dysfunction related to urination, defecation, and sexual activity. This pain and dysfunction can occur in both men and women. One person may experience only one symptom while another may experience all symptoms. Symptoms vary, as do their anatomical locations, yet we propose that the trigger for these symptoms may be the same and a common effective treatment may exist for all of them.

Not something you talk about at a party

Even though many people suffer from *a headache in the pelvis*, most of them feel alone in their difficulty. The genital, urinary, and defecation areas are considered private and are often very difficult to talk about, even with close friends or relatives. Basically, we want the areas of the genitals and rectum to work, but we don't want to know much about them, or to have to pay any attention to them.

These areas of the body are not treated with much respect. This is a truth that is reflected in how we word profanities. What do we call people at whom we are angry? Usually terms related to defecation or procreation are used in a derogatory way. Indeed, these are terms of denigration. In our culture, the genitals and rectum are shrouded in shame and guilt. As we discuss later, the genitals and rectum are areas that are often psychologically and energetically disowned by people. Being rejected in some way, it is not uncommon for people to distance themselves physically from these body parts by tightening against them. The healing of the abused pelvis, as Steven Levine has stated eloquently, in part involves bringing the genitals and rectum "back into the heart." This means changing one's attitude from shame, guilt, and rejection to compassion and appreciation.

People's aversion toward these areas can be so strong they will often go to the doctor only when the symptoms are marked. Sometimes they dismiss these symptoms as aging or as normal aches and pains that have to be tolerated. Sometimes people will endure symptoms for long periods of time, if they can bear them, because they are afraid that if they seek a diagnosis, it will be one that they don't want to hear. They prefer not to know. Given the embarrassment about these areas, the anxiety over what symptoms can lead to, and the poor treatment record of the medical profession, it is not surprising that sufferers of chronic pelvic pain syndromes often feel isolated.

The confusion of names

An old parable to explain a current confusion

Once upon a time, ten blind men, each with a cane, went for a walk along a road that skirted a jungle. Soon they came upon an elephant, and each one found himself at a different place in relationship to the animal. One blind man touching the elephant's leg remarked, "Oh, this creature is like a tree trunk." Another, who was positioned under the elephant's stomach, pushed up and said, "Oh no. This creature is like a soft ceiling, with nothing else around on the sides." A third positioned at the tail, pulled on it and said, "No, this creature is like a rope connected to a tree." Another, touching the trunk of the elephant, said, "No, this creature is like a large, soft pipe." Yet another, reaching and touching the elephant's tusk, said, "No, this creature is like a curved spear stuck into rock."

On and on they argued. What was this creature they had come upon? Finally, a fellow traveler came by and heard the argument. Noticing right away they were blind, he said, "No, you're all correct, and you're wrong, because this is an elephant and each one of you is only touching one part, thinking that each part constitutes the whole."

For reasons about which we can only speculate, up to the present day, the manifestations of chronic pelvic pain syndromes have been perceived by blind men. This is not to disparage the sincere physicians who grapple with these conditions. It is, however, in the nature of the specialization of medicine, that physicians only see a problem through the lenses of their own field, and depending upon the specialist you see, the condition may be called by a different name.

What might be called prostatitis by an urologist might be called *coccygodynia or pudendal nerve compression* syndrome by a colorectal surgeon. Other names used by specialists to describe the same condition are *chronic genital pain, prostatodynia, essential anorectal pain, idiopathic pelvic pain, pelvic floor myalgia, spastic piriformis syndrome,* and others.

Similarly, what might be called *vulvar vestibulitis, lichen sclerosis, lichen planas, or lichen simplex chronicus* by a dermatologist might be called a yeast infection by a gynecologist, or an anxiety disorder by a psychiatrist. If you go to three doctors for chronic pelvic pain, it is easily possible you can get two or three different diagnoses.

One important reason for this "blindness around seeing the whole elephant" is the lack of communication among the many medical specialties. If they all spoke to each other and shared information, they might realize they often are talking about the same condition. It is the hope of the authors of this book that we can bring eyes to bear on this problem that have a broader scope. We aspire to see the whole elephant.

General Symptoms of Chronic Pelvic Pain Syndrome in Men

Intermittent or constant pain

For both sexes, all of the symptoms described below can either be intermittent or constant, diurnal or nocturnal (daytime or nighttime), during sitting or standing and often more profound during periods of stress. Symptoms can involve pain and no urinary or sexual dysfunction, pain and urinary symptoms with no sexual symptoms or all three. One of the perplexing aspects is the variable cycles of intensity.

In men, chronic pelvic pain includes *pain in the rectum* or perineum, between the scrotum and anus. Patients report that it feels as if there was a "golf ball" there. Often symptoms include *pain when sitting.* Many men experience pain in the area above the pubic bone in and around the area of the bladder, called *suprapubic pain. Pain in the groin* is typical and can be experienced unilaterally or bilaterally (on one side or both sides). Pain in the testicles called *orchalgia* is not uncommon. *Pain in the penis* is often felt at the penile tip or in the urethra. Sometimes there is *coccygeal pain* (in or around the tailbone), or *pain in the lower back* or, not uncommonly, *thigh pain* in the back, side, or front of the thigh, either on one side or both.

Intermittent or constant urinary symptoms in men

Disturbances in urination are often associated with pelvic pain. Commonly with pelvic pain, men experience something called *dysuria,* which is pain, discomfort, or burning when urinating. They also complain of a *reduced urinary stream, frequency of urination* (in which they have to urinate every half hour to two hours), *urgency of urination* (in which they feel they can't wait to urinate once the urge arises), and/ or *nocturia* (a need to urinate frequently at night).

Intermittent or constant sexual dysfunction in men

Sexual discomfort, during or after ejaculation, is sometimes associated with pelvic pain. Commonly, men complain of a *reduced libido* or desire for sex and sometimes erectile dysfunction (occasional or frequent inability to attain or maintain an erection). Sometimes the pain of ejaculation acts as a deterrent to sexual desire.

Intermittent or constant psychological symptoms in men

Almost universally, men experience *anxiety* and various levels of low spirits or *depression*. They have the sense that "there's something wrong inside me." It is not unusual for men to complain of *dysphoria*—to have a reduced interest in participating in life and in interpersonal relationships. Some degree of withdrawal from social situations occurs and self-esteem often suffers.

General Symptoms of Chronic Pelvic Pain Syndrome in Women

Intermittent or constant pain

In women, the symptoms described can be either intermittent or constant. As with men, women can experience pain or related dysfunction more during the night or during the day, more in the morning or in the afternoon, more during or not during their menstrual cycle, and often more during periods of stress.

Location of pain in women

Women can experience genital pain in the form of *vaginal/vulvar pain* (pain at the opening of the vagina or deep inside). In certain conditions, women experience *coccygeal pain* (pain at the tailbone) and *rectal pain* (pain at the opening or inside the rectum). In other conditions, women, like men, report *suprapubic pain* (pain right above the pubic bone, in and around the area of the bladder), *groin pain, and pain when sitting.* Some women complain of pain in the *sub-pubic region*, including *pain in the clitoris.*

Intermittent or constant urinary symptoms in women

Urinary symptoms may coexist with many conditions of pelvic pain. Women can experience *urinary frequency, urinary urgency, dysuria, reduced urinary stream, and incomplete bladder emptying.*

Intermittent or constant sexual dysfunction in women

Because there is often *vaginal pain* at the opening or inside the vagina, *dyspareunia* (pain during or after intercourse) is almost always present. In more severe cases, particularly with women who have *vulvar vestibulitis*, there is an *inability to have intercourse*. This may be their only complaint.

Intermittent or constant psychological symptoms

Given the nature of the symptoms of these conditions, it is easy to understand why feelings of *anxiety* and depression are sure to follow. Because of the part of the body that is involved, and the severe impact on the ability to be sexual, an *impairment of intimate relationships* occurs with many women. Women may lose their zest for living. Generally, the more pronounced and constant the symptoms, the more severe the dysphoria. Naturally, the self-esteem of many women who suffer from these conditions tends to be low.

Symptoms Listed Related to the Traditional Diagnostic Categories

In the following section, we will introduce the name that has been traditionally used for a certain pelvic pain syndrome, followed by a simple explanation of what the name means. We will then summarize the symptoms that are traditionally included under this name, the number of people affected by the condition, the traditional treatments used, and how helpful or unhelpful they are. Following this, we will discuss in more detail the symptoms and the condition in general.

Prostatitis

Category I – Acute Bacterial Prostatitis

Description

Acute Bacterial Prostatitis is quite clear both in its diagnosis and in its treatment. Infection and inflammation are evident and traditional treatments work well. We do offer the idea that chronic pelvic tension may be its initiating cause.

It can occur at any age and manifest with symptoms such as fever, chills, pain, and urinary dysfunction. Positive findings involving the presence of white blood cells in the urine confirm this diagnosis. Acute bacterial prostatitis develops relatively quickly and is often associated with a feeling of being sick. Newer antibiotics produce good results. It is important to have this condition treated quickly because of the risk of the spread of bacteria into the bloodstream, retention of urine, and potential abscess formation. Chronic bacterial prostatitis can develop from acute bacterial prostatitis that is poorly treated. Antibiotic therapy should be extended to 28 days to assure eradication of the infection.

Symptoms

- Fever and chills
- Prostate pain
- Dysuria
- Lower back pain
- Perineal pain (pain between the anus and scrotum)
- Difficulty urinating
- Urinary retention

Because of retention of urine due to swelling of the prostate gland, a catheter may be inserted into the penis to allow for proper flow of urine. While this catheter may increase the risk of prostatic abscess or infection in the gland, catheterization is an important part of therapy when there is urinary retention. Some men with acute urinary retention may be better served with a small plastic catheter inserted directly into the bladder through the skin of the suprapubic area.

Factors associated with onset

- Migration of bacteria up the urethra
- Unprotected anal intercourse
- Immune disorders
- Urinary retention or instrumentation

Prevalence

- Approximately 5% of reported diagnoses of prostatitis (relatively rare)

Tests for Diagnosis

- Urinalysis (microscopic inspection)
- Culture of urine (important and often neglected by physicians)

Traditional treatments used

- Antibiotics (muscle injection of aminoglycosides or penicillin, oral fluoroquinolones)

Success of traditional treatment

- The most successfully treated type of prostatitis

Category II – Chronic Bacterial Prostatitis

Description

Chronic Bacterial Prostatitis represents a more difficult condition than acute bacterial prostatitis. Most chronic bacterial prostatitis develops because of inadequately treated acute prostatitis. Men who have recurrent bacterial colonization of the urethra because of poor hygiene, poor sexual practices, or a need to instrument the urethra may have bacterial colonization and infection. Men who have strictures or scar tissue in the urethra that narrow the tube restricting urinary flow may be prone to developing recurrent bacterial infection. Often there is no bacterial growth in the bladder and one can be completely asymptomatic between episodes of acute flare-up, at which time the bacteria grow, spread, and begin to infect the bladder. This is a hallmark of chronic bacterial prostatitis. Men are usually free of symptoms between "attacks."

Symptoms (may be intermittent or constant)

- Urinary frequency (need to urinate more than every two hours)
- Dysuria (pain or burning during urination)
- Recurring urinary tract dysfunction with poor flow, hesitancy, and nocturia (frequent voiding at night). These symptoms also mimic enlargement of the prostate gland.
- Symptoms are intermittent depending on the bacterial burden. In an individual, repeated "attacks" tend to be associated with the same bacteria.

Factors associated with onset

- Inadequately treated acute bacterial prostatitis
- Calculi or stones in the prostate
- Uncircumcised, with poor hygiene

Prevalence

- Approximately 5% of all men who have prostatitis (relatively rare)

Tests for diagnosis

- Localized urinary and prostate fluid cultures are very important but often neglected by physicians
- Positive bacterial localization from prostate during periods with no symptoms

Traditional treatments used

- Fluorouinolone antibiotics have proven to be the most effective, usually requiring a minimum of six weeks of therapy
- Nitrofurantoin can suppress flare-ups of infection but does not eradicate the organism
- Occasionally, because of enlargement of the prostate with age and the occurrence of multiple stones in the prostate, a patient may benefit from transurethral resection of the recurrently infected tissue

Success of traditional treatment

- Antibiotics are usually effective for acute flare-ups
- Eradicating recurrent episodes is difficult. Antibiotics used for this condition may become less effective over time because the bacteria may mutate and become resistant

Category III – Chronic Nonbacterial Prostatitis
(sometimes with inflammation IIIA, or without inflammation IIIB)

Description

Chronic Nonbacterial Prostatitis represents by far the largest number of cases of men who bear the general category of prostatitis. It has been estimated that this category involves 90-95% of all cases diagnosed as "prostatitis." In terms of numbers in the United States, this condition affects tens of millions of men at some time in their lives. Recent research has increasingly pointed out that conventional ideas and treatments for nonbacterial prostatitis have simply failed to both explain and treat the problem. Traditional approaches have treated this kind of prostatitis as an infection, although in recent years, doctors have acknowledged their befuddlement about the cause and cure of this condition. In 1995, the National Institutes of Health, in a consensus conference on prostatitis, acknowledged that the terms *chronic nonbacterial prostatitis* and *prostadodynia,* neither explained nor were even related to the symptoms. A new name was then adopted for this condition: *chronic pelvic pain syndrome (CPPS).* In changing the name of the most common disorder seen by urologists, there was the clear implication that the prostate could not necessarily be indicted as a cause of this disorder.

Studies have shown that men undergo severe impairment in their self-esteem and their ability to enjoy life in general because the pain and urinary dysfunction is so profoundly intimate and intrusive. The effect on a person's life with nonbacterial prostatitis has been likened to the effects of having a heart attack, having chest pain (angina), or active Crohn's disease (bleeding/inflammation of the bowel). If nonbacterial prostatitis moves from a mild and intermittent phase to a chronic phase, sufferers tend to live lives of quiet desperation. Having no one to talk to about their problem, usually knowing no one else who has it, and receiving no help from the doctor in its management or cure, they often suffer depression and anxiety.

Symptoms (may be intermittent or constant and include one or more of the following)

- Pain in the rectum (often described as a "golf ball" in the rectum)
- Suprapubic pain (pain above the pubic bone)
- Perineal pain (pain between the scrotum and anus)
- Pain in the penis
- Coccygeal pain (pain in and around the tailbone)
- Low back pain (on one side or both)
- Groin pain (on one side or both)
- Dysuria (pain or burning during urination)
- Nocturia (frequent urination at night)
- Urinary frequency (need to urinate often, usually more than once every two hours)
- Urinary urgency
- Reduced urinary stream
- Sense of incomplete urinating
- Hesitancy before or during urination
- Pain or discomfort during or after ejaculation
- Reduced libido (reduced interest in sex)
- Anxiety about having sex
- Anxiety in general
- Depression
- Social withdrawal and impairment of intimate relations
- Impairment of self esteem

Nonbacterial prostatitis is a condition that produces much suffering. There are no curative drugs or effective surgical procedures. Experimental treatments have been attempted and have also failed. These treatments include acupuncture, reflexology (foot acupressure), magnetotherapy (magnets inside the rectum), optical-quantum-generator radiation therapy, rectally-administered ultrasound, bee pollen, corticosteroids, mud therapy, intrarectal electrical stimulation, saw palmetto (herb), and zinc (mineral).

What is often more troubling to men who have this condition than their actual physical symptoms are the depression and discouragement that comes from their helplessness to do anything about their condition. Many doctors are less than enthusiastic to treat nonbacterial prostatitis because they know that they have very little to offer the patient. This often leads patients to feel that no doctor gives them any time or consideration when they seek help for this problem.

Furthermore, it is common to see high levels of anxiety in men with nonbacterial prostatitis because of their fear that their symptoms indicate they have cancer or some undiagnosed disease.

The desperation of men with this condition leads some of them to find doctors who do heroic and unwarranted kinds of interventions. In our clinic we have seen patients who have had resection or removal of prostate tissue or years of antibiotics, all in the service of "doing something" about the problem.

Factors associated with onset (may include one or more of the following)

- High periods of stress
- Weight lifting
- Pelvic surgery
- Anxiety-producing sexual encounter
- Trauma to the pelvis
- Bacterial prostatitis
- Compulsive sexual activity or masturbation
- Prolonged sitting at work

Prevalence

- It has been estimated that up to 50% of all men at some time in their lives (in U.S., tens of millions) suffer from this condition.

Tests for diagnosis

- Absence of significant bacteria as determined by culturing and counting load from the prostatic secretion. This requires laboratory bacterial culture
- Microscopic analysis of prostatic fluid to determine the presence of white blood cells or inflammation. This category may involve inflammation or be completely without inflammation
- Analysis of urinary bladder and pelvic floor behavior utilizing physiologic testing (urodynamics) such as urine flow rate, retention of urine, measurement of bladder pressure, and nerve activity
- Digital rectal examination and prostate serum enzyme to rule out cancer or other abnormalities of the prostate
- Transrectal ultrasound (TRUS) may be beneficial to evaluate the image of the prostate and sperm storage organs (seminal vesicles), but most importantly to perform prostate biopsies in the event of abnormal blood tests or palpation

Traditional treatments used

- Antibiotics almost always given whether or not there is a sign of infection
- Prostate massage
- Adrenal nerve blocking agents (alpha blockers) to relax the smooth muscle of the prostate and bladder neck
- Low dose antidepressants (low doses of Elavil®)
- Muscle relaxants/tranquilizers (Valium®; antidepressants such as Prozac® or Paxil®)

Success of traditional treatment

- Antibiotics generally not useful
- Prostate massage occasionally gives symptomatic relief, but is of limited effect
- Alpha blockers (Hytrin®, Cardura®, Flomax®) sometimes give limited symptomatic relief but may have high levels of adverse side effects

- Muscle relaxants/tranquilizers, especially benzodiazepines such as Valium®, offer some temporary reduction in pain but because of side effects and tendency towards dependence, are not useful as a main-line treatment

Category IV– Asymptomatic Prostatitis

Description

Asymptomatic Prostatitis can be thought of as a 'sleeper condition' in that a man will not recognize he has it because there are no subjective symptoms. Usually it is discovered when a man sees a doctor who finds evidence of inflammation through either a biopsy or examination of prostatic fluid under a microscope. This is a significant condition because there is evidence that inflammation of the prostatic fluid or semen may cause a rise in the PSA level (prostate specific antigen), which is routinely screened now in men over 50 and thought to be an indicator of possible prostate cancer. When men eliminate infection through antibiotic treatment, the PSA level returns to normal, and the concern about cancer is removed. Diagnosing this condition therefore eliminates the need for further testing for prostate cancer including prostate biopsy. PSA also usually rises in proportion to enlargement of the prostate gland.

Symptoms (may be intermittent or constant)

- No subjective symptoms for patient
- Increased level of white cells in prostatic fluid or semen
- PSA often elevated (prostate specific antigen that sometimes indicates prostate cancer when elevated)

Factors associated with onset

- Unknown

Prevalence (number of people)

- Number unknown. This condition is poorly understood, and is usually only detectable through PSA screening or prostatic fluid analysis

Tests for diagnosis

- Elevated PSA
- Indications of inflammation in the prostatic fluid/semen

Traditional treatments used

- Four weeks of antibiotics

Success of traditional treatment

- Unknown

A Headache in the Pelvis in Women

Vulvodynia (Vulvar Vestibulitis, Dysesthetic Vulvodynia)

Vulvar vestibulitis is a syndrome that is marked by pain at the opening of the vagina when touched. There are women who have vulvodynia who only have pain when the vulva is touched and at no other time. As a result, many women who suffer from this simple kind of vulvodynia have pain during intercourse or simply cannot have intercourse. Many cannot wear tight clothing or engage in any activities that put pressure on the opening of the vagina.

The other kind of vulvodynia is called dysesthetic vulvodynia. This is a more challenging condition because it involves chronic pain and a sense of burning in the vulva whether the vulva is touched or not. Dr. Howard Glazer, the psychologist who discovered the usefulness of biofeedback for this condition (which we will discuss in Chapter 3), has found that simple vulvar vestibulitis syndrome is associated with abnormally high tension in the muscles of the pelvic floor. Dysesthetic vulvodynia, on the other hand, seems to be connected with pelvic floor muscle weakness.

Symptoms (may be intermittent or constant and women may have one or more of the following symptoms)

- Pain when the opening of the vagina is touched
- Pain during intercourse
- Erythema (redness of tissue at the bottom of the opening of the vagina)
- Chronic pain (dysesthetic vulvodynia)

Women with vulvodynia often end up seeing a number of doctors before they receive the correct diagnosis. Gynecologists have often confused vulvodynia with a yeast infection. They then prescribe treatments for a yeast infection which aggravate rather than help the condition. In a way, this is not unlike the man who sees the urologist for pelvic pain and is reflexively given antibiotics.

Dermatologists are also consulted for this problem and have had little to offer. Patients sometimes go to a dermatologist because vulvodynia appears to be a problem involving the skin, but treatments of the skin have rarely proven helpful.

As has happened with many conditions for which the cause is unclear, numerous alternative and fringe treatments have emerged. Modifications of diet (including elimination of foods with oxalates, chocolate and caffeine), acupuncture, reflexology (foot acupressure), and analgesic creams are among some of the treatments offered for this problem. Neither the traditional treatments nor the alternative/fringe treatments have offered much help.

Factors associated with onset (may include one or more of the following)

- Chronic yeast infections and the use of antifungal agents sometimes associated with onset
- Often no obvious associated factors
- Higher incidence is associated with sexual trauma (rape, sexual abuse)

Prevalence

- Approximately 16% of women sometime in their lives

Tests for diagnosis

- Patients report intermittent or constant pain and/or burning at the opening of the vagina upon touch.
- Severe tenderness to a cotton swab that brushes over the opening of the vagina
- Dyspareunia (pain during intercourse)

Traditional treatments used

- Surgery
- Topical estrogen creams
- Psychotherapy

Success of traditional treatment

- Surgery is controversial with very inconsistent results
- Topical creams have little effect upon symptoms
- Psychotherapy is also used, but is generally not useful in reducing symptoms

Urethral Syndrome

Urethral syndrome is another condition that affects women and has not been well understood or treated. Women with urethral syndrome often complain of one or several of the following symptoms: dysuria, a sense of straining in order to urinate, urinary frequency, urinary urgency, hesitating at the commencement of and during urination, incontinence, and suprapubic pain. The symptoms can be either intermittent or constant, and they tend to wax and wane. It is our view that in many cases, interstitial cystitis (inflammation of the bladder lining) has been misdiagnosed as urethral syndrome.

Symptoms (may be intermittent or constant)

- Dysuria (pain during urination)
- Urinary frequency (the need to urinate with abnormal frequency)
- Urinary urgency (an urgent need to urinate with little ability to postpone urination)
- Hesitation during urination
- Incontinence (the inability to hold in urine)
- Suprapubic pain (pain above the pubic bone)

While urethral syndrome tends to resolve itself without treatment after a period of time, there are women who seem to have this problem chronically. Sometimes alleviation of symptoms occurs after dilation of the urethra using a thin metal rod, although there is considerable controversy about this method in medical circles. When this procedure does not help and the physician is unable to detect any obvious physical problem, the woman who suffers from urethral syndrome often has to deal with her exasperated doctor who may label her condition as a psychiatric one. Psychotherapy, as with almost all conditions of pelvic pain, tends not to be helpful in its resolution.

Factors associated with onset

- Unknown

Prevalence

- Unknown

Tests for diagnosis

- Patients report of urinary frequency, urgency, hesitancy, incontinence
- Suprapubic pain (pain above the pubic bone)

Traditional treatments used

- Antibiotics
- Urethral dilation (inserting a metal rod into the urethra with the intention of stretching it)

Success of traditional treatment

- Antibiotics tend not to be helpful
- Urethral dilation does help some women

A Headache in the Pelvis in Both Men and Women

Interstitial Cystitis and Painful Bladder Syndrome

Interstitial cystitis (IC) has been a controversial diagnosis. Some doctors even believe it does not exist as a separate entity. Other doctors are clear about the existence of IC as a separate and distinct disorder caused by inflammation of the bladder.

Common symptoms of IC include suprapubic pain and perineal pain. Dyspareunia is often reported by women who have this problem. Some foods, such as those considered spicy, as well as alcohol and caffeine, seem to exacerbate symptoms. Urinary frequency and burning discomfort in the urethra are present in almost all cases of IC. We have seen patients who have had to urinate as often as four times an hour, day and night.

The frequency of urination plays havoc with routine activities. Sufferers have to go to the bathroom very frequently during work, when they're attending a conference or a concert, and during the myriad of other activities that require one to be able to comfortably hold urine for reasonable periods of time. Urinary frequency often seriously disturbs sleep.

People with IC tend to report a history of urinary tract infections. In IC, however, the inflammation of the bladder that is believed to be the cause of the symptoms of IC is not the same as the inflammation that one finds with an ordinary urinary tract infection that can be treated with antibiotics.

Interstitial cystitis used to be thought of as a "woman's disorder." Today, while most cases of IC affect women, men have been diagnosed with it as well. The estimate is that out of the approximately five hundred thousand to one million people who are affected by IC in the United States, 88% of the sufferers are women, and 12% are men. However, these estimates represent only the 20% of sufferers who have been diagnosed.

People with IC often have other problems. It has been observed that some women with IC also may have fibromyalgia and vulvar vestibulitis as well. IC tends to be more prevalent among Jews and less common among African-Americans. There may be associated bowel discomfort sometimes diagnosed as irritable bowel syndrome as is often the case with most of the conditions of pelvic pain that we discuss.

While no treatments at this time are curative, a number of treatments do exist that can sometimes reduce symptoms. One common treatment which is also a diagnostic method for IC consists of cystoscopy under anesthesia with bladder hydrodistention. This means that one is put under general or regional (spinal) anesthesia, and a tube is inserted into the bladder with a video camera assisting the view and allowing pictures of the lining of the bladder after the bladder is pumped full of water. If the tissue or urothelial lining tends to break and bleed after releasing the pressure, it is suggestive of a chronic inflammation. This procedure alone, however, sometimes alleviates the symptoms for a while after the procedure pain has passed.

In a study that throws some question on this standard test for IC, however, women who had no symptoms of IC underwent cystoscopy under anesthesia with hydrodistention of the bladder. A considerable number had bleeding in their bladders when dilated in the same way as women who complained of IC-like symptoms. These women, however, reported having no pain and no symptoms. This observation has cast some doubt on the standard procedure to diagnose IC. If there are people who have sensitive and fragile bladders but complain of no symptoms whatsoever, the question arises as to whether the sensitive and fragile bladder is in fact the cause of the suffering of IC. There is evidence that half of the people with IC symptoms spontaneously get better with no treatment at all. Furthermore, research in Scandinavia revealed that the source of IC pain was not found in the bladder, but mostly in the muscles of the pelvic floor.

Symptoms (may be intermittent or constant)

- Urinary frequency (the need to urinate more than once every two hours)
- Pain during urination (as well as before or after urination)
- Suprapubic pain (pain above the pubic bone), presumed to be bladder pain
- Some patients report dietary sensitivity (spicy foods, alcohol, chocolate, caffeine) while others do not
- Fragile bladder wall (as seen in cystoscopy under anesthesia)
- Perineal pain (pain between the scrotum and rectum in men, and between the vagina and rectum in women) and penile pain in men
- Dyspareunia in women (pain during and after sexual intercourse)

Factors associated with onset *(may include one or more of the following)*

- Occasionally acute bladder infection
- Usually factors seem to be unknown

Prevalence

- Approximately one million people in the United States (90% women, 10% men)

History for diagnosis

- Patients report of urinary frequency (the need to go to the bathroom very frequently or more than once every two hours on a regular basis)
- Patients report of urinary urgency (the subjective sense of an urgent need to urinate)
- Patients report of increase of symptoms with spicy foods, alcohol, chocolate, and caffeine
- Ulceration, mucosal tearing, glomerulations (microhemorrhage with distention) in several places in the bladder
- Hypersensitivity to a potassium solution put in the bladder

Traditional treatments used

- Elmiron® (pentosan polysulfate, a medicine partially secreted in the urine to assist coating the bladder surface)
- Elavil® (amyltripiline, an antidepressant to suppress the pain fiber response)
- Antihistamines to combat mast cells that secrete stimulating biochemicals (histamines)
- Bladder instillations that infuse medication like DMSO (a solvent type product derived from wood) directly into the bladder—may be accompanied with cortisone and heparin

- Bladder stretching (pumping water directly into the bladder to stretch it)
- Modifications in diet involving elimination of foods that seems to increase symptoms

Success of traditional treatment

- Most treatments help some people some of the time
- Self-help efforts like diet modification and smoking cessation tend to reduce symptoms
- No procedure thought to cure

Levator Ani Syndrome

In the 1950's the term *levator ani syndrome* was used to describe a disorder that involves a high degree of pain in the rectal area. Both men and women can suffer on either an intermittent or constant basis. When sufferers are in constant pain, sitting can make it worse. For those with intermittent pain, it can be set off by sitting, standing, or lying down. Some patients also complain of constipation. It is estimated that the majority of these patients are women, and that this condition seems to affect people at midlife.

When a digital-rectal examination is performed, pain is elicited by pressing on a small area within the levator ani muscle. When the doctor sweeps his finger from back to front along the muscle, it feels like a tight band. Often, though not always, the tenderness is on one side.

Levator ani syndrome is rarely associated with urinary or ejaculatory symptoms. While proctologists (doctors who specialize in disorders of the colon and rectum) naturally tend to see patients with levator ani syndrome, gastrointestinal doctors, urologists, and physical therapists also see such patients.

In recent years, a small group of urologists have diagnosed what has been called levator ani syndrome as pudendal nerve compression syndrome. This controversial viewpoint theorizes that the source of rectal pain derives from the compression of the pudendal nerve. Nerve blocks and surgery to presumably decompress the pudendal nerve are advocated by these urologists. The results of these treatments of nerve blockade and surgery have been very mixed. There is no published research that documents the efficacy of such procedures and, perhaps more important, documents the substantial risks of these treatments. These risks include the destabilization of the pelvis as the result of cutting the sacrotuberous and sacrospinal ligaments as well as increased chronic and possible permanent pain that was not present before this surgery.

It is not uncommon for patients with levator ani syndrome to see many doctors and travel great distances in the hope of relief. A number of different approaches have been used for this problem. Some doctors have attributed the condition to poor posture and have educated the patient on how to sit in a less stressful way, although poor posture as a cause of levator ani syndrome remains speculation. In the middle 1930's, a series of studies reported success in digitally massaging the tight levator ani muscle. Later in the 1950's and 1960's, others also reported some degree of success doing this.

Electrical stimulation (inserting a steel probe in the rectum and running an electrical current into the rectal muscles) has been used by a number of physicians with varying degrees of success.

Biofeedback, in which a probe is inserted into the rectum and hooked to a sensitive machine that feeds back to the patient slight degrees of tension in the external muscles of the anal sphincter, has also been used with varying degrees of success.

Symptoms (may be intermittent or constant)

- Intermittent or constant rectal pain
- Absence of abnormal physical findings

Factors associated with onset (may include one or more of the following)

- Constipation in some patients
- Increased level of tension at the opening of the anus
- Reduced strength of the external anal muscles

Prevalence (number of people)

- Majority are female
- Absolute numbers unknown

Tests for diagnosis

- Patients report of rectal pain
- Pain elicited when pressing levator ani muscle in rectum
- Absence of urinary symptoms
- Absence of ejaculatory or post-ejaculatory discomfort

Traditional treatments used

- Reassurance to patient that no life-threatening illness is found
- Electrical stimulation sometimes used
- Ultrasound sometimes used
- Biofeedback sometimes used
- Hot baths
- Tranquilizers, muscle relaxants
- Anti-inflammatory medications

Success of traditional treatment

- Reassurance to patient that no life threatening illness is found is useful and relieving but not curative
- Electrical stimulation sometimes used with varying degrees of usefulness
- Ultrasound sometimes used with results unclear
- Biofeedback sometimes used with some studies reporting success

- Hot baths often temporarily reduce symptoms
- Tranquilizers and muscle relaxants temporarily reduce symptoms
- Anti-inflammatory medications have unclear results

The assumptions underlying the conventional medical understanding

As we will discuss, one of the most important factors in the treatment of any condition is your understanding of what it is in the first place. In the next chapter, we will present the existing conventional ideas of chronic pelvic pain syndromes while making explicit the often unspoken assumptions upon which they rest.

CHAPTER 2

THE OLD MODELS AND TREATMENTS

*"It's not a good idea to do open heart surgery
if the problem is heartburn."*
Anonymous

*"The answer to an unsolved problem is rarely
found in the field designated to study it."*
Martin Schwartz, Ph.D.

The way you see a problem is the key to solving it

In the nineteenth century, Ignaz Semmelweiss, a Hungarian physician, sought to discover the cause of what in his day was called *puerperal fever,* a horrific malady that took the lives of many young pregnant women and the children they bore. While this scourge was known throughout the history of medicine, its occurrence was relatively uncommon. This usually rare malady reached epidemic proportions in the European hospitals of the seventeenth, eighteenth and nineteenth centuries. Indeed, the "fever," that was a streptococcal infection, would now be considered the result of unconscionably bad hygiene. It occurred almost exclusively in the crowded hospitals of the urban areas of Europe.

The physicians in the large hospitals of France, Germany, England, and Ireland could not figure out why so many women died of the puerperal fever. A number of theories explaining the fever were popular at the time. They included the beliefs that it came from a discharge of the uterus, from the accumulation of milk inside the body of the mother, from gastric biliousness, from the emotions of fear and shame, from an increase in fibrin in the bloodstream of the mother and from influences of the weather. Considering what we understand about hygiene and infections now, these ideas seem preposterous, but they were part of the accepted lore explaining the deaths from the fever.

Semmelweiss painstakingly investigated the illness. Several clues pointed him toward viewing the fever as an infection caused by poor hygiene. He noticed that women, who gave birth outside the hospital, usually because they were giving birth to illegitimate children, rarely got the fever. He concluded that the problem was to be found within the hospital itself.

Secondly, Semmelweiss noticed that a close friend of his, whose work included dissecting cadavers during anatomy classes, became sick and died after he cut himself with the knife that he was using to dissect a cadaver. His symptoms appeared identical to those of women who had died of the *fever*. From this and other evidence, Semmelweiss concluded that unwashed particles from the dissection of cadavers and from surgery on infected patients were entering the bodies of the pregnant women.

With this understanding, Semmelweiss devised a protocol for doctors and other caregivers. It involved making the environment as clean as possible for the delivering mother. This included always washing the hands with a mixture of lime juice and chlorine as an antiseptic.

While it is hard for us to understand how people could object to such a protocol, one that simply insisted upon cleanliness and frequent hand washing in and around the hospital, Semmelweiss in fact came up against great opposition. There were vicious attacks upon his proposals, attacks which brought about much suffering in his life. Among his detractors was his immediate boss and supervisor, a Dr. Klein, who blocked and hampered him at every turn. Klein was not the only one. Semmelweiss had to deal with many opponents, even though the efficacy of his efforts appeared indisputable.

As we examine Semmelweiss's situation now, it appears that his supervisor, Dr. Klein, may have been threatened by Semmelweiss's vigorous campaign to reform the hygienic habits in the hospital. Klein may have felt that Semmelweiss was indicting him for the deaths of women who contracted puerperal fever.

In his biography of Semmelweiss, Frank Slaughter observes that *when a new idea is introduced, it is usually first met with rejection and repudiation by forces in medicine that are invested in maintaining the old way.* Only after time passes and the efficacy of the new idea is established, is the advance accepted.

Medical knowledge and treatment is always a work in progress. The world of pelvic pain research and treatment is no different. Some practitioners are invested in a certain way of looking at this problem, and they resist any change, especially if the new methodology fails to depend upon their expertise and/or does not benefit them economically.

If we are in hot water long enough, we forget we are hot and wet

As we see in the case of Semmelweiss, it is difficult to dislodge old assumptions. People often don't even know they have them. *When frogs are placed in warm water and the temperature is gradually increased to the boiling point, the frogs remain in the water and boil to death. On the other hand when a frog is immediately placed in hot water, it immediately jumps out.* Most of us are 'swimming' in the old ways of thinking and don't even know we are wet.

Our way of thinking defines a problem and it dictates the kind of solutions that are possible. In the Middle Ages, for example, the concept of disease was that it was caused by four humors being out of balance. Consequently, it would make sense to treat disease with blood letting, purging, and vomiting, since it was believed that such maneuvers purged and rebalanced the system. We gradually discovered over time that this way of thinking is not based on fact and that it severely limited the effectiveness of treating illness. Our concepts of disease and medicine have evolved, and new and more efficacious approaches have been the result.

Changing our ideas of disease alters the way we treat it. On an individual level, *your notions about what is wrong with you determine what you will do to help yourself.* In modern times we have discarded the idea that illness is caused by humors. None of us would consider bloodletting or purging to improve our health. It is equally important, however, to be clear today about the thoughts and assumptions we hold about pelvic pain that motivate our choice of treatment.

Does the old way of thinking empower the patient or stimulate fear and helplessness

Fifty years ago, two gastroenterologists who did research at medical center near New York conducted an experiment to show the effect of one's mental picture of a bodily condition on the condition itself. These researchers did rectal examinations of naïve male subjects. Looking up the rectum of a subject, one of the two doctors present would casually say to the other, within earshot of the subject, that something looked cancerous inside the rectum. The other doctor would agree and then they would observe what happened in the subject's colon. The researchers reported that commonly the colon of the subject would go into an immediate spasm. As soon as the doctors reassured the subject that he was healthy and did not have cancer, the spastic colon immediately released. This experiment illustrated how a catastrophic idea about your health can have an immediate and profound effect.

Negative and catastrophic thinking palpably increase pain in those with pelvic pain. Many of the men we see with prostatitis are, at some level, worried they have cancer or some other life-threatening disease. It is not uncommon for patients with pelvic pain to walk around for many years carrying catastrophic thoughts relating to their pain that, as we will discuss later, exacerbate their pain and greatly impoverish the quality of their lives. The reassurance that what they have is not life-threatening can sometimes alleviate their symptoms on a short-term basis. More important than our reassurance, however, is teaching the patient to manage his or her own negative thinking as well as contraction of the pelvic floor.

The power of trust, reassurance and the placebo effect

A placebo is commonly thought of as a sugar pill, essentially a substance with no known medically active ingredient that helps a patient's symptoms. It is thought that the power of the placebo derives from the patient's belief that the pill will help. It is this trust that the substance will make everything okay that is the key ingredient in the placebo's power.

When you talk about the placebo effect, you are talking about the effect of feeling with complete certainty that "you are going to be completely okay, everything is fine, it will all be taken care of, don't worry, or fret at all, forces larger than you love you and will make sure you are safe, sound, and happy." The placebo effect = everything-is-going-to-be-okay effect. The placebo effect is the great antidote to anxiety and fear. The placebo, with regard to our condition, returns us to being carefree as children are carefree. No anti-anxiety drug can equal the power of the real placebo effect.

The power of placebo attests to the power of a *thought* reassuring someone that they are safe and everything will be okay. The power of placebo indirectly attests to the power of fear to disturb both body and mind because placebo simply acts to remove fear and doubt.

The communication of this thought also appears to be the chief ingredient in the power of a good doctor's bedside manner. In the presence of such a doctor, the patient's anxiety dissolves in the idea that all will be well again. This is not unlike a child's trust that his loving parents will take care of him.

If you are experiencing pelvic pain or discomfort now and the anxiety and contraction that usually comes with it, imagine that someone were to say to you "We will take care of this. You will be completely healed and back to normal." Notice what effect this might have on your symptoms. Many people with pelvic pain experience a reduction or sometimes even an abatement in symptoms on a short-term basis as the result of trying something new that they think will help them. This is the placebo effect.

It is agreed that there is a substantial placebo effect with *any* treatment for chronic pelvic pain. We believe that the short-term relief people with a nonbacterial condition obtain from antibiotics is primarily the result of the placebo effect. In the second printing of our book, we reported on a published study that scientifically validates our long held position. Ciprofloxin®, one of the most powerful of antibiotics, on a long-term basis proves to be only as effective as a placebo.

The power of placebo is not small. A dramatic example occurred with a man who suffered from pelvic pain for ten years. He reported he entered a doctor's office in a great deal of pain. The doctor, whom the patient described as kindly and confident, felt this patient's prostate gland and said "Your prostate is completely normal. Our test revealed no evidence of anything wrong. You are completely healthy down there. Go out with your wife and have a night on the town and celebrate your good fortune." The man reported he left the doctor's office with no pain. Moreover, he remained pain-free for months, even though it gradually returned. There is no known medicine that can alleviate pelvic pain for months. This illustrates that the placebo effect and the trust that everything will be okay, on a short-term basis, has the ability to loosen the knot of chronic tension and anxiety that binds the contents of the pelvis.

The letting go of tension afforded by a placebo is analogous to *the letting go that is the focus of our treatment*. However, placebos only work as long as the person either consciously or unconsciously believes the problem has been solved. The difference between our treatment and a placebo, as we shall discuss, is that we actively assist the patient in restoring the patient's *ability* to voluntarily relax the pelvis and the thinking associated with its chronic tightness.

In our culture, the doctor is thought to understand the true reality of the patient's mental and physical state. Typically, patients with pelvic pain adopt the doctor's viewpoint of their condition and they adopt the implications of the diagnosis as well. The doctor's diagnosis can add to a sense of fear and foreboding that patients already carry with them. A doctor's suggestion that prostatitis may be an autoimmune disorder, for example—a suggestion that is simply an educated guess with little data to support it—can easily scare patients who are already confused. Many doctors lose sight of how much their ideas communicate to patients. An offhand comment that a doctor makes to a patient can either haunt or relieve a patient for years.

A Stanford psychiatrist found that women with breast cancer who participated in support groups lived significantly longer than those who did not. This was startling information and demonstrated the profound positive impact of social/psychological factors in creating disease on the one hand and extending life and well being on the other.

What you name what is wrong with you can hurt you or help you

If the positive thought of knowing that there is a place to share your deepest feelings can enhance both the quality and length of life, so too can adverse thoughts injure us. A number of researchers have found that the *diagnosis* of cancer itself can traumatize individuals. Studies have shown that some people who have been diagnosed with cancer subsequently exhibit signs of post-traumatic stress disorder. These signs do not derive from the physical presence of cancer but from the terror that the diagnosis triggers.

It is not difficult to understand why the diagnosis of cancer is a traumatic event. Imagine what it would mean to your life if a doctor told you had cancer. Your life would invariably change as the shock of the diagnosis settled in. Even if you had no physical symptoms, the diagnosis alone would shake you to your foundation. *What you call what is wrong with you can clearly hurt you or help you.*

Before we see patients, we ask them to fill out a form in which they score their pain and urinary dysfunction levels. In the past, this sheet was titled "Chronic Pelvic Pain Symptom Score" and its purpose was to establish the person's experience of his or her condition. When we first developed the form, no attention was given to the effect of the title on the patient. In light of our discussion, we see that patients had to confront the term *chronic pelvic pain* and identify themselves as chronic sufferers every time they came into the clinic.

The term *chronic* means ongoing and continual, implying that the condition will not go away. We came to realize that the title of the form might be causing levels of unnecessary suffering. While our patients' pain may have been chronic in the past, we could not say with certainty that their pain or dysfunction would not go away in the future. We changed the name of the sheet to "Pelvic Pain Score."

We saw that *a diagnosis almost always implies a prognosis.* Why would any caring doctor want to use a diagnosis that sentenced someone to a depressing future when such a negative outcome is in no way a certainty? Our title, *A Headache in the Pelvis*, reflects our compassionate interest in discussing these difficult conditions in a credible way that does not condemn people to such dismal future outcomes. Indeed, our title reflects our optimism for the possibility of a successful resolution of the problem.

Limitations of the Old Model

When you view your body as a machine

When we see a doctor, the nurse often puts us in a small, windowless room where we wait on an examining table or sit on a chair. We busy ourselves reading a magazine until we hear the door open and the doctor enters. He talks to us for a few minutes, perhaps examines our body, and then gives us a piece of paper, which we take to the pharmacy. When all goes well, and after a few pills, the complaint is resolved.

We take for granted that the doctor usually does not talk to us about our thoughts, feelings, home situation, sex life, or spiritual practices. We assume it is normal for the doctor to be interested only in the specific problem for which we are in the office, a problem with our body. Furthermore, we take for granted that the actual time spent with the doctor will probably be a few minutes or less.

We know that modern medicine typically looks at the body as a machine. However, the implications of that view are profound and far-reaching. If the body is a machine, it is a thing, an object, a piece of meat. The body, in some profound way, is not considered to be conscious, to have any intelligence, or to be something to which one has to listen carefully.

When the body is seen as a machine, one searches for the defective part to be fixed. An illustration of this is found in the treatment of vulvar vestibulitis. Doctors observe redness at the bottom of the vagina, which the woman reports as tender. For some physicians, the solution to this problem has been to surgically remove this red and irritated tissue. In our experience, the results have largely been ineffective.

In our practice, we have seen patients whose prostates have been removed, whose pelvic muscles have been surgically severed, whose bladders have been removed, whose testicles have been removed, whose pelvic nerves have been dissected and whose pelvic stabilizing ligaments have been severed—all in the service of getting rid of the part of the body/machine that is thought to be the source of the problem. The patients we have seen who have undergone such medical care have most often not been helped by such interventions, and more often have had to endure greater suffering, not only from the original source but from the surgical interventions.

The rest of the person, including his way of thinking, his emotional state, his life style, values—things that are not measurable—tend to have only secondary importance in the doctor's office. When the doctor examines the patient and can find no part of the body the doctor specializes in that appears to be causing the problem, the doctor often concludes that the problem is mental. To the patients we have seen, this kind of diagnosis has been invalidating and depressing and the treatments they have undergone for the so-called 'mental' condition have routinely failed to help their problem.

In treating your painful pelvic floor from the current body-as-a-machine perspective, it is as if the doctor were saying to your pelvic floor:

"You must have been invaded by bacteria or are inflamed for some reason. I am going to use drugs to get rid of this bacteria or inflammation. Your pain is something that shouldn't be there. It is not informative. It shouldn't be considered or listened to. It is not saying anything. Your pain and dysfunction has no relation to how your owner is thinking, feeling, working, being in relationship, or generally living his or her life and I have neither the time for nor the interest in how you might be part of the larger picture of your owner's life. Considering the larger picture of your owner's life and how that might help you is a foreign idea to me. I am simply interested in silencing you. If I do that, I have been successful in my work."

When the doctor brings this viewpoint to the suffering of someone with a chronic pelvic pain syndrome, the patient often adopts the following kind of view of his or her own pelvic floor:

"I feel your burning, pain, tightness, soreness, or rawness and I am afraid of you. The doctor wants to get rid of you but can't get rid of these sensations. He doesn't seem to know what's wrong with you. Whatever I try to do does not get rid of you. You might mean terrible things. You may mean that I can never have health, happiness, joy, love, relationship, parenting, and fulfillment in my life. You shouldn't be here. You are a mistake, an error and a defect in me. You have nothing to say to me. You are bad. Whenever I feel you, I feel afraid and discouraged. I want to get as far away from you as possible. I hate you and want to get rid of you."

Your body wants to heal

The old medical model views the body as composed of modular parts that can be replaced or repaired when defective. This modular model seems to dismiss the notion that the body has intelligence and consciousness and that it can heal itself.

Dr. Dean Ornish pioneered a treatment that derives from a dynamic and functional way of understanding the body. He offered a treatment for individuals with heart disease, which put them on a low fat diet, taught them yoga, and provided them with group support. He discovered that, following this multifaceted regimen, the blocked state of their arteries reversed.

Dr. Ornish demonstrated the truth that *the body has the intrinsic capability of regenerating and healing itself under the right conditions.* By intrinsic, we mean that this ability for regeneration and self-healing is part of the very nature of the body. In the healing process, the challenge is to learn how to provide the best environment for healing to occur.

Nowhere is the dynamic and intelligent nature of the body more visible than in the effects of exercise. Sit in a chair without moving for three or four weeks and your muscles atrophy. Your heart muscle will actually diminish in size because the requirement for pumping blood has been reduced. Those who have been bed-ridden for a prolonged period know all too well the effect of no exercise on muscle tone and strength and general well-being.

All of us have observed that when we cut ourselves, clean the wound, and put a band-aid over it, a miracle occurs. In a number of days, the cut is healed. Most of us take this miracle for granted and simply expect this stunning intelligence of the body to do its own healing. If a car that was damaged in a car accident could gradually fix a dent or scrape all by itself we would be stunned.

We know the cut does not need our conscious effort or direction to heal. The healing is intrinsic, natural, and in the very nature of tissue. There is however, a condition necessary for the healing to occur. One must give the cut an environment within which it can heal. Pick at it, allow dirt and bacteria to enter it, and it won't heal. The key is to understand what the requirement for healing is and make it a reality. This is obvious for some conditions and not so obvious for other conditions. In the past, when human beings did not understand that microbes that were invisible to the eye could enter a wound and infect it, they often failed to make the kind of environment needed for their healing.

Healing is a word that is seldom used in the discussion or treatment of chronic pelvic pain syndromes. At the time of the second printing of this book, in the National Library of Medicine, in over 5000 medical research studies on the chronic pelvic pain syndromes discussed in this book, the word healing occurs only 11 times. In our book, we are proposing that to treat pelvic pain and dysfunction one must first understand what the pelvis needs for its own healing. *We are proposing that the key to healing, in general, and the resolution of certain kinds of pelvic pain and dysfunction in particular, involves learning skills that will free the healing potential in the body.*

Appreciate the intelligence of your body; see your symptoms as your body trying to talk to you in the form of pain and dysfunction

When you appreciate the intelligence of your body and see your symptoms as your body trying to talk to you, you take a different viewpoint from the one resulting from the conventional medical model. From this viewpoint, it is as if you are saying to your pelvic floor, "I feel your burning, pain, tightness, soreness, or rawness and it doesn't feel good to me and I know it doesn't feel good to you. I know you want to feel better and be out of pain. I know you are happiest when you function properly. I know that you wouldn't be complaining this way without a reason. I know you want to heal. I want to understand what you are saying to me in your pain and dysfunction and listen to how I can help you. I want to regard you like my own child who does not feel well, who can't speak to tell me what is wrong, and who needs my compassion, love, unconditional presence, and help. I don't want to separate myself from you but instead I want to stay close to you as a loving parent would stay close to his or her unhappy child. I am here for you without condition and will do whatever I can to lovingly make an inner home for you so that you can get better. I care about you."

Such a viewpoint brings about joining and not separation between you and your pelvic floor. It brings an attitude of peace and understanding to your pain and dysfunction. It does not wage a war. Such an attitude relaxes and does not tighten. It sees the sore area of the pelvis as an inarticulate friend in need and not an enemy. It brings love and not hate, integration and not separation, compassion, understanding and not fear.

A man who recovered from pelvic pain by using our protocol reported an experience that illustrates how bodily symptoms represent a language the body is using. Here is his story.

"I did not have any problem with my teeth for quite a while. I was brushing regularly and my dentist told me my gums reflected the good care I was taking of them. One day, out of the blue, I noticed that my upper molar was exquisitely tender. I was dismayed. I thought that I was doing such a good job with my teeth. Whenever I would go to the dentist, it would always cost many hundreds of dollars. I dreaded the pain, the expense, and the time in having to go yet again. I was also anxious about what it might mean about the strength of my teeth given that this pain was happening in the midst of the best care I could give myself.

Discouraged, I picked up the phone and dialed my dentist's office. The receptionist quizzed me as to what the problem was and where the location of the pain was, and suggested that I come in for the dentist to check my teeth. In the middle of making this appointment, I poked around the painful area of the tooth and felt a little piece of toothpick lodged there. I told the secretary to hold the line as I dislodged the end of a toothpick that was stuck in between the teeth.

To my amazement the pain suddenly stopped. I asked the secretary if a piece of toothpick lodged in between teeth could cause pain and she answered yes. I told her that I had just dislodged this piece of toothpick and that I was going to cancel the appointment I had just made because perhaps I had found and solved the problem.

I realized that the pain in my tooth was the only way the tooth had to tell me there was something wrong. The pain was not arbitrary or vindictive. It was simply the language of my body. I realized that I usually don't listen to my body's language, especially when there is pain. I usually get frightened by this kind of bodily communication and run to ask someone to reassure me that I am okay.

The suddenness with which the pain stopped brought home to me the intelligence and sincerity of my body. It was telling me that something was stuck in my tooth that needed to be removed. I felt like apologizing to my tooth for my distrust of the pain, and for not understanding that the pain was my friend and not my enemy."

In our view, pelvic pain is no different from the tooth pain described above. It represents the pelvis trying to talk to us and tell us that something needs correction. The primary pain does not intend to generate fear. *The purpose of the pelvic pain we treat is to notify us that something needs attention so it can heal.*

The Old Way of Treating Prostatitis

Over the last fifty years, the viewpoint that has emerged to explain what prostatitis is and what its treatment should be derives from the idea that prostatitis is an infection and/or inflammation of the prostate gland. Indeed, that's what its name indicates, that it is an "itis" of the prostate.

When a man comes into the physician's office and complains about pelvic/urinary/rectal/genital pain and/or urinary symptoms like frequency, urgency, dysuria (pain during urination), if there are no physical findings, the picture that comes into the doctor's mind almost exclusively is that the prostate gland has a bacterial infection or that there is an inflammation. Even today, prostatitis is seen as an infection or inflammation often without any tests to establish the validity of such a diagnosis. As we have seen in a study of physicians in Wisconsin, a large majority of doctors view prostatitis as an inflammation or bacterial infection, and almost all prescribe antibiotics as a treatment. Most urologists know from their own experience that antibiotic treatment for prostatitis without evidence of inflammation or infection routinely fails to resolve the patient's symptoms and yet almost 100% of the cases of this kind of prostatitis receive antibiotics.

The treatment of *bacterial prostatitis* with antibiotics has been an achievement of modern medicine. *Viewing all conditions of pelvic pain and dysfunction in men as acute or chronic bacterial prostatitis is erroneous. Despite the clear scientific evidence to the contrary and every urologist's clinical experience of the ineffectiveness of antibiotics for nonbacterial prostatitis, it is amazing that giving antibiotics for nonbacterial prostatitis is in keeping with the current standard of care of medical practice. This is very important to understand, particularly if you have been diagnosed with abacterial prostatitis.* Urologists are trained rigorously in the skills of the surgeon. The narrow focus on a part of the body that is defective and needing surgical intervention or drugs is also, in large part, the focus of these doctors. Furthermore, many surgically-trained doctors scoff at the intimation that prostatitis-like pelvic pain involves the relationship between the body and the mind and that both body and mind need to be addressed in treatment. The idea that anxiety, negative thinking, sexual practices, work habits, environment, and interpersonal relationships must be addressed in treating certain pelvic pain dysfunctions is something about which most urologists feel less than enthusiastic.

The system of reimbursing the doctor for his services contributes powerfully to the way the patient is treated as well as contributing to the maintenance of the general view of the problem. Several doctors have confided to us that their prostatitis patients are the most difficult, complain the most, and are the patients for whom insurance companies reimburse the least. Indeed, in the minds of most physicians, we believe there is very little financial incentive to explore what else might be going on in the life of the person who has prostatitis or in the relationship between his mind and his body.

While the old way of thinking clearly has failed to explain or help the conditions we discuss in this book, it remains in place in the practice of medicine throughout the United States. A patient comes in to the doctor's office complaining of prostatitis, the doctor does some tests, diagnoses the problem as prostatitis, and gives the patient an antibiotic. This is problematic because certain kinds of antibiotic therapy can have serious long term detrimental side effects especially when there is no reason for such treatment.

Drug companies and resistance to changing medical thinking

The major drug and medical equipment companies, which are an important source of funding for medical research in America, tend not to favor supporting alternative non-drug or non-surgical treatments for pelvic pain. The focus of their research efforts lie in developing new drugs and medical equipment, the sale of which will allow their companies to financially prosper. This economic reality supports the continued use of the traditional methods of treatment and perpetuates the paradigm that only drugs or surgical procedures are the answer to chronic pelvic pain disorders.

New Forces for Change

To reiterate, most doctors who treat nonbacterial prostatitis know that they have very little success using antibiotics for this condition. At the same time, they continue to prescribe them.

Dr. Lawrence True, a pathologist at the University of Washington Medical School, took multiple biopsies of the prostates of 97 men who complained of pelvic pain and symptoms of prostatitis. He found that in 95% of the cases, there was no evidence of clinically significant infection or inflammation. Furthermore, he found there was no correlation between evidence of inflammation or infection in the prostatic fluid and any inflammation or infection in the tissue of the prostate. He concluded that the evidence suggested that researchers look elsewhere to determine the cause of prostatitis symptoms.

In our experience at Stanford, we find that symptoms are most severe with "prostatitis" patients who have *no evidence of infection or significant inflammation.*

The growing demand for answers: the power of the internet

In the past few years, the internet has become a major force for change in many areas, including traditional thinking about prostatitis and chronic pelvic pain syndromes. Prior to the internet, it was common for a man with prostatitis to see a urologist, be given antibiotics that failed to help, and then fade away out of medical view to simply suffer with his symptoms.

Not so anymore. Now, the sufferer of prostatitis, receiving no help from his doctor, goes to the internet to find other avenues or advice to deal with this problem. This is now true for all medical conditions. The popularity of websites offering medical information is a testimony to this. The ability to search for alternative medical opinions and treatments on the internet represents a profoundly important change in medicine. The doctor has ceased to have the last word.

The rise of patient advocate organizations

The internet has made it possible for sufferers to form support groups. No matter how obscure the medical condition, one can go easily onto the "net" and find an appropriate group.

The information accessible on the prostatitis website is not confined to traditional viewpoints held by most doctors. Viewpoints that patients would never have heard about ten years ago now coexist along with the traditional ideas. It has been suggested that the webmaster may ultimately be more influential in medicine than the doctor by democratizing the exposure of different viewpoints that otherwise would not have been made available to patients.

The word 'prostatitis' is 'googled' thousands of times per month. The Prostatitis Foundation (www.prostatitis.org) and the Chronic Prostatitis website (www.chronicprostatitis.com) have thousands of people per month accessing their websites for information. When you consider that it takes an educated and sophisticated individual to do a search on the internet and even to spell the word "prostatitis" correctly, it is not unreasonable to assume that the real size of the population of sufferers exceeds this number. As the internet grows, and as it becomes more commonplace for ordinary people to have access to it, we will likely see the power of these organizations increase.

Examining the Limitations of the Old Way of Thinking About Chronic Pelvic Pain Syndromes

When we examine the old ideas, the limitations become obvious. When doctors train to become specialists, the assumptions underlying the old way of thinking about chronic pelvic pain syndromes are rarely discussed. The doctors-in-training adopt these assumptions as a way of becoming members of the specialist's club. Below we ask a series of pointed questions about the old way of looking at and treating chronic pelvic pain syndromes. These questions relate to the issue of whether the old ideas about chronic pelvic pain syndromes see the body as a machine, and whether they see any relationship between body and mind, lifestyle, intimate relations, work environment, sexual behavior, spiritual life, patient responsibility, and the healing of pelvic pain.

The body as a machine

Does the medical viewpoint regard the body as a machine and symptoms as a sign that the parts need to be replaced or repaired? Is the body viewed as an unintelligent object and the disorder compartmentalized, simply requiring that the problematic part be fixed?

Acute bacterial prostatitis

- Yes

Chronic bacterial prostatitis

- Yes

Chronic nonbacterial prostatitis, with or without evidence of inflammation

- Yes

Asymptomatic inflammatory prostatitis

- Yes

Proctalgia fugax

- Yes

Interstitial cystitis

- Yes

Levator ani syndrome

- Traditionally, the syndrome involves rectal pain with unknown origin

Vulvodynia (vulvar vestibulitis)

- Yes

Urethral syndrome

- Yes

Body and mind

Does the medical viewpoint include a connection between body and mind? Is the condition seen as some event related to a person's mental and emotional life?

Acute bacterial prostatitis

- No

Chronic bacterial prostatitis

- No

Chronic nonbacterial prostatitis, with or without evidence of inflammation

- No

Asymptomatic inflammatory prostatitis

- No

Proctalgia fugax

- No

Interstitial cystitis

- No

Levator ani syndrome

- No

Vulvodynia (vulvar vestibulitis)

- Sometimes regarded as a psychiatric disorder

Urethral syndrome

- No

Lifestyle

Does the medical thinking take into account any connection between the condition and the patient's lifestyle? By lifestyle, we refer to whether someone is living alone or with others, whether they have pets, whether they have hobbies, what kind of work they do and their feelings about it and their sexual orientation.

Acute bacterial prostatitis

- No

Chronic bacterial prostatitis

- No

Chronic nonbacterial prostatitis, with or without evidence of inflammation

- No

Asymptomatic inflammatory prostatitis

- No

Proctalgia fugax

- No

Interstitial cystitis

- No connection to lifestyle except for diet

Levator ani syndrome

- No

Vulvodynia (vulvar vestibulitis)

- No

Urethral syndrome

- No

Intimate relationships

Does the medical thinking see any relationship between the patient's condition and his intimate relationships? Is he married, and if so, what is the state and quality of the relationship? What is the relationship with family? Does he or she have friends? Does he or she feel connected to others or isolated?

Acute bacterial prostatitis

- No

Chronic bacterial prostatitis

- No

Chronic nonbacterial prostatitis, with or without evidence of inflammation

- No

Asymptomatic inflammatory prostatitis

- No

Proctalgia fugax

- No

Interstitial cystitis

• No

Levatora ani syndrome

• No

Vulvodynia (vulvar vestibulitis)

• No

Urethral syndrome

• No

Work environment

Does the medical thinking see any relationship between a person's work and condition? How does patient feel about his work? Is it a pressure cooker requiring 100 hours per week or an easy job? Does he or she have a boss with whom the patient gets along or does he or she feel oppressed by the boss? Is the job sedentary or active?

Acute bacterial prostatitis

• No

Chronic bacterial prostatitis

• No

Chronic nonbacterial prostatitis, with or without evidence of inflammation

• No

Asymptomatic bacterial prostatitis

• No

Proctalgia fugax

- No

Interstitial cystitis

- No

Levator ani syndrome

- No

Vulvodynia (vulvar vestibulitis)

- No

Urethral syndrome

- No

Sexual behavior

Does this viewpoint see any relationship between a person's sexual life and practices and the condition of the pelvis? Is he or she sexually active? Does the patient masturbate and if so how frequently? What goes on during sex in terms of a person's level of relaxation or tension?

Acute bacterial prostatitis

- No

Chronic bacterial prostatitis

- No

Chronic nonbacterial prostatitis, with or without evidence of inflammation

- No

Asymptomatic bacterial prostatitis

- No

Proctalgia fugax

- No

Interstitial cystitis

- A person with IC often has pain during sex when symptomatic

Levator ani syndrome

- No

Vulvodynia (vulvar vestibulitis)

- No

Urethral syndrome

- No

Spiritual life

Does this way of thinking see any relationship between a person's spiritual life and the condition of his or her pelvis? Does the patient have a spiritual interest or spiritual practice? Is there any comfort or distress in his life as a result of his or her spiritual beliefs or practice?

Acute bacterial prostatitis

- No

Chronic bacterial prostatitis

- No

Chronic nonbacterial prostatitis, with or without evidence of inflammation

- No

Asymptomatic bacterial prostatitis

- No

Proctalgia fugax

- No

Interstitial cystitis

- No

Levator ani syndrome

- No

Vulvodynia (vulvar vestibulitis)

- No

Urethral syndrome

- No

Patient responsibility

Does the physician assume the sole responsibility for the patient's healing or does he view the patient equally responsible?

Acute bacterial prostatitis

- Only insofar as patient must take medication

Chronic bacterial prostatitis

- No

Chronic nonbacterial prostatitis, with or without evidence of inflammation

- Only insofar as the patient must take medication

Asymptomatic inflammatory prostatitis

- Only insofar as the patient must take medication

Proctalgia fugax

- No

Interstitial cystitis

- Traditional model sees management of diet sometimes helpful for symptom relief

Levator ani syndrome

- No

Vulvodynia (vulvar vestibulitis)

- No

Urethral syndrome

- No

Empowerment or fear and helplessness

Does the viewpoint itself empower the patient, imply, or specifically state measures that can be taken to resolve the condition, or does the perspective leave the patient feeling afraid and helpless?

Acute bacterial prostatitis

- Empowers patient because antibiotics usually stop the symptoms

Chronic inflammatory prostatitis

- Both empowers and encourages helplessness. Empowers if antibiotic stops symptoms. Encourages helplessness if episodes recur.

Chronic nonbacterial prostatitis, with or without evidence of inflammation

- Tends to create fear and helplessness because therapy is ineffective; the model does not correspond with most patients' experience

Asymptomatic inflammatory prostatitis

- Empowers

Proctalgia fugax

- Empowers

Interstitial cystitis

- Viewpoint in part tends to encourage fear and helplessness in that no cure is offered

Levator ani syndrome

- Encourages fear and helplessness, as the traditional approach does not understand the condition and there is no agreement upon effective treatment

Vulvodynia (vulvar vestibulitis)

- Encourages fear and helplessness, as there is no effective cure

Urethral syndrome

- Encourages fear and helplessness, as there is no effective cure

Cause

What is the essential element (according to the conventional medical thinking) that causes the condition?

Acute bacterial prostatitis

- A bacterium

Chronic bacterial prostatitis

- A bacterium

Chronic nonbacterial prostatitis, with or without evidence of inflammation

- Immune disease

Asymptomatic inflammatory prostatitis

- A bacterium

Proctalgia fugax

- Muscle spasm

Interstitial cystitis

- Probably immune disorder

Levator ani syndrome

- Unknown

Vulvodynia (vulvar vestibulitis)

- Unknown

Urethral syndrome

- Unknown

Cure

What is the essential element (according to the conventional medical thinking) that brings about resolution or cure of the condition?

Acute bacterial prostatitis

- An antibiotic

Chronic bacterial prostatitis

- An antibiotic

Chronic nonbacterial prostatitis, with or without evidence of inflammation

- An antibiotic, anti-inflammatory agent, alpha nerve blocker

Asymptomatic inflammatory prostatitis

- An antibiotic

Proctalgia fugax

- Unknown

Interstitial cystitis

- Traditional treatments can sometimes alleviate symptoms, but no cure is offered

Levator ani syndrome

- None

Vulvodynia (vulvar vestibulitis)

- None

Urethral syndrome

- Stretching the urethra

Treatments

What are the treatments that are used in the conventional model?

Acute bacterial prostatitis

- Oral antibiotics

Chronic bacterial prostatitis

- Oral antibiotics

Chronic nonbacterial prostatitis, with or without evidence of inflammation

- Oral antibiotics
- Prostate massage
- Sitz baths
- Dietary recommendations – avoiding alcohol and caffeine
- Zinc tablets
- Recommendations to increase frequency of ejaculations
- Alpha blockers (Hytrin®, Cardura®, Flomax®)
- Antidepressants (Elavil®)
- Muscle relaxants (Valium®)
- Non-steroidal anti-inflammatory agents

Asymptomatic inflammatory prostatitis

- Oral antibiotics

Proctalgia fugax

- None

Interstitial cystitis

- Elmiron® (a medication which attempts to help restore a competent surface mucosa to the lining of the bladder)
- DMSO bladder instillation (infusing DMSO and other substances in the bladder to alleviate inflammation)
- Bladder behavior modification (bladder drill)
- The patient is asked to increase the time between urinations in order to stretch the bladder
- Immune therapy using tuberculosis vaccine in the bladder (BCG)
- Antidepressants (Elavil®)
- Antihistamines
- Electrical stimulation neuromodulation

Levator ani syndrome

- Electrical stimulation
- Ultrasound treatment
- Hot baths

Vulvodynia (vulvar vestibulitis)

- Surgery in certain cases
- Topical estrogen creams
- Low oxalate diet

Urethral syndrome

- Urethral dilation that includes inserting a metal rod in the urethra and stretching it

Efficacy

How effective are the treatments used within the conventional model?

Acute bacterial prostatitis

- Very effective

Chronic bacterial prostatitis

- 70%-80% are symptom-free after effective antibiotic therapy

Chronic nonbacterial prostatitis, with or without evidence of inflammation

- All traditional treatments are largely ineffective
- Antibiotics that permeate the prostate are not effective
- Dietary modifications are not effective when bladder is not involved
- Prostate massage can give occasional temporary symptomatic relief
- Zinc tablets and saw palmetto berry are not effective
- Increased ejaculations are not effective
- Alpha blockers sometimes provide relief, often have distressing side effects, and are not curative

Asymptomatic inflammatory prostatitis

- Unknown

Proctalgia fugax

- Not effective

Interstitial cystitis

- Traditional treatments sometimes alleviate symptoms

Levator ani syndrome

- Varying degrees of success are reported with treatments listed. Levator ani syndrome is not seen to have a known cause or cure in traditional practice
- Generally a low level of efficacy with conventional treatments

Vulvodynia (vulvar vestibulitis)

- Surgery sometimes has good results with certain kinds of vulvar pain, while other times surgery is claimed to have bad results with more and symptoms
- Topical estrogen creams have reported minimal effects
- Psychotherapy has reported minimal effects
- Generally a low level of efficacy with conventional treatments

Urethral syndrome

- Urethral dilation is sometimes effective but remains a controversial treatment

CHAPTER 3

A NEW UNDERSTANDING OF CHRONIC PELVIC PAIN SYNDROMES LEADS TO AN EFFECTIVE THERAPY

Summary of Our Understanding

We have identified a group of chronic pelvic pain syndromes that we believe are associated with the overuse of the human instinct to protect the genitals, rectum, and contents of the pelvis from injury or pain by contracting the pelvic muscles. This tendency becomes exaggerated in predisposed individuals and over time results in chronic pelvic pain and dysfunction. The state of chronic constriction creates pain-referring trigger points, reduced blood flow, and an inhospitable environment for the nerves, blood vessels, and structures throughout the pelvic basin. This results in a cycle of tension, anxiety, and pain, which has previously been unrecognized and untreated.

Understanding this tension, anxiety, and pain cycle has allowed us to create an effective treatment. Our program breaks the cycle by rehabilitating the shortened pelvic muscles and connective tissue supporting the pelvic organs while simultaneously using a specific methodology to modify the tendency to tighten the muscles of the pelvic floor under stress.

It is our belief that the chronic pelvic pain syndromes may begin with a person's habit of focusing tension in the muscles of the pelvis. This tendency sets the stage for the disorder. What triggers the symptoms can be a major stress or several minor stresses occurring simultaneously. The stressors can be psychological or physical. Once set off, anxiety and protective bracing fuel pain and dysfunction and a self-feeding cycle begins that seems to have a life of its own.

The reason that chronic pain and dysfunction resist a simple mechanical fix is that they tend to come out of a background of a life-long habit of focusing tension in the pelvic muscles. It is necessary to rehabilitate the pelvic muscles in conjunction with changing the predisposition to pelvic tensing under conditions of stress.

In order to make our understanding clear, we offer the allegory below followed by a step-by-step analysis of the story. We advise our readers to take time to read the allegory as it will help clarify their understanding.

An Allegory

Once upon a time, there was a land called the pelvic floor upon which the whole world depended for its survival and pleasure. The pelvic floor provided vital services for the world including filtering and eliminating wastes, providing sexual pleasure, and helping structurally support the world in its various activities. The land of the pelvic floor performed these services best when its citizens lived a life of balance between work and rest.

It came to pass that the world went through a period of strife, and the citizens of the pelvic floor were required to work more and more. Night shifts became common place. In some parts of the land, citizens were required to work twenty four hours a day, seven days a week, with no rest.

Soon the pelvic floor citizens were completely exhausted and very unhappy. They had stopped doing their jobs well. Their normal processing of wastes was no longer done efficiently, and they became able to give little pleasure to the world. Their cries of distress were increasingly heard.

Painful protests from the pelvic floor were made with demands for a return to the balance between rest and work. The world, however, did not seem to understand what the pelvic floor was trying to say.

So the world hired a consultant who suspected the source of the problem to be foreign troublemakers and recommended sending in legions of anti-troublemakers. The troublemakers, however, could not be found and the problem continued.

The world became desperate and decided to hire a new consultant who saw the problem differently. The new consultant said, "If you want to solve this problem, you must go to the land of the pelvic floor and listen to its complaints." The world replied, "We don't know how to talk to or understand the pelvic floor. We have never had a conversation with it." The consultant answered, "I know the language of the pelvic floor and will teach you how to understand what it is trying to tell you."

After meetings with the pelvic floor and the consultant, the world finally understood that its contribution to the problem was the demand it made for the pelvic floor to work constantly. So the world decided to change this. However, while the world agreed in principle to stop demanding constant work, it often forgot this agreement and lapsed back into its old habit of making unreasonable work demands. The consultant had to remind the world over and over to stop forcing the pelvic floor to work constantly. This was not easy for the world to learn.

After a while, the world said to the consultant, "Your method seems to be working much of the time but why is everything not completely back to normal?" The consultant replied, "Both you and the land of the pelvic floor are used to the unhappy state of affairs. If you are not reminded, you will continue to force the citizens of the pelvic floor to work without rest."

The world, however, was not the only perpetuator of the problem. The pelvic floor had also gotten used to the misery of constant work and had forgotten how to rest even when the world allowed it.

Therefore, a curriculum was set up for the pelvic floor as well. The people of the pelvic floor went to special clinics where they learned to stretch the contracted posture that they developed due to their constant work. This stretching and their lessons in learning not to fall back into the old habits enabled them to relearn how to relax and rest.

As the world and the pelvic floor learned to coexist in a balance of work and rest, the land of the pelvic floor became a happy place again.

Pelvic pain and dysfunction associated with overused and chronically tensed pelvic musculature

In our allegory, the world stands for you, the conscious person, who makes decisions and sends commands to your body. You send these commands, often out of habit. They feel normal and familiar to you.

The pelvic floor is your pelvis and the contents of your pelvis including the structures that are involved in urination, defecation, sexual activity, and physical movement. These functions and their myriad of biochemical, nervous, and mechanical processes go on often without requiring your awareness, will, conscious effort, or attention.

We see in the allegory that the problem begins when the world demands that the pelvic floor work on a constant basis. Normally, the pelvic floor muscles are dynamic, working, and resting throughout the day. Even though they tighten, they have the ability to relax. The relaxed state allows for proper oxygenation, nutrition, management of wastes and rejuvenation of tissue.

The pelvic floor muscles are not meant to be chronically contracted. When muscles are chronically tensed, they tend to shorten and eventually accommodate so that the posture of a shortened state of the muscles feels normal.

People who have pelvic pain syndromes tend to habitually focus tension in the pelvic muscles as a response to stress, anxiety, trauma, or pain. In our allegory, we allude to this by saying that the continual strife of the world prompted it to make the pelvic floor work too much.

The tendency to focus tension in the pelvic muscles is not an accident. *Some have suggested that a person's inclination to focus tension in the pelvic muscles begins with toilet training. The child is able to stop his parent's reaction to soiling by tightening his pelvic muscles. Over time, tightening the pelvis becomes a conditioned reaction to any situation in which anxiety arises.* Let us be clear that this idea of focusing tension in the pelvic muscles as a result of early toilet training is simply an idea and we do not propose that it should be taken as fact. It is however, a compelling explanation of how pelvic tension may well begin early in life. Other thoughtful investigators such as Tony Buffington, a veterinarian, also imply that neuroendocrine patterns may be formed early in life to create susceptibility to pain pathways.

Research has shown, and it is our clinical experience as well, that people with chronic pelvic pain syndrome tend to have elevated pelvic floor tension even when resting. The pain and dysfunction gets worse in the presence of stress. Most of our patients notice this relationship between stress and the severity in their symptoms. This observation leads to the heart of our understanding.

In our allegory, we see that the constant demand made upon the pelvic floor leads to a disruption in its ability to function. It is our view that, over time, a constant demand on the pelvic floor to tense results in an environment that is inhospitable to the nerves, blood vessels, and structures within it. The pelvic floor is not made of steel and in certain individuals is quite disturbed by chronic tension.

It is our view that the person who has the kind of pelvic pain we discuss in this book has sore and irritated pelvic tissue. This tissue is not viewed by conventional medicine as pathological. We believe that this sore, shortened, contracted tissue is a very real physical condition. People who have chronic pelvic pain feel this soreness and irritation acutely. It sometimes feels like a burning, aching, tightness, tearing or a very sore area of what feels like raw tissue. When the doctor or physical therapist trained in *Myofascial/Trigger Point Release* feels the inside of the rectum or vagina in patients with chronic pelvic pain syndrome, he or she often reports feeling areas of restriction and areas of tension and taut bands (trigger points) which, when touched, cause patients to jump with pain. Some professionals who work inside the pelvic floor of people with pelvic pain describe the tissue as *gunky* or *rock-like*. Areas within the pelvic floor which have been subjected to years of continual contraction need time to heal even when the muscles are no longer under tension. When physical therapy is properly done, and the pelvic floor is regularly rested, what feels like gunky, rock-like tissue often becomes soft, supple and pain free.

The painful pelvis is like a continually contracted fist

Imagine tightening your fist as hard as you can for an hour. You notice that there are places of lighter color in your hand that result from squeezing the blood out of the blood vessels. Your hand will feel uncomfortable and you feel relieved to stop the squeezing.

Now imagine you maintain this clenched fist for a day. Now imagine you maintain this fist for a week. Now imagine a month of tightening your fist constantly twenty-four hours a day. Now imagine doing it for a year. Now imagine doing it for several years. This is one way to understand the state of the pelvic floor in people with pelvic pain.

Imagine, after several years, you stopped tightening your fist. Do you think the great discomfort and irritability of the tissues of your hand would immediately stop? Almost certainly not. It is not hard to imagine that you would want to rub your hand, massage it, take each finger, and stretch it out to relieve it from the contracted state it had been in. Nor would it be hard to imagine that, even after you stopped tightening your fist, your fist would still be sore. It would take some time, some pampering, and most importantly, no chronic retightening of the fist before your hand felt normal again.

Imagine continually tensing your pelvis

Chronically tightening your fist is one thing. Now imagine you were asked to tighten your pelvic muscles for 30 seconds as if you were stopping yourself from urinating. For most people this pelvic tightening would not be the most pleasant thing to do but it would be doable. Imagine you tightened up in the pelvis like this for a minute. It would still be doable. Now imagine you were asked to keep your pelvic muscles continually tensed for 30 minutes… now 1 hour… now 6 hours... now 12 hours… now 24 hours… now 1 week... now 1 month… now 1 year… now 2 years… now 5 years.

People who have never had pelvic pain are incredulous at being asked to contract their pelvic muscles for 30 minutes. The prospect of continual tightening of the pelvic muscles for a week, month, or year would be unthinkable and yet the research shows increased tone in the pelvic floor for many people with pelvic pain. Dealing with such a condition is the focus of our protocol.

In our allegory, the consultant the world first chose refers to the traditional physician who routinely assumes the presence of infection as the source of the difficulty (foreign troublemakers). But, treating these troublemakers, or the presumed bacteria, has failed to resolve the problem of chronic pelvic pain syndromes. Recent research has shown antibiotics to be no more effective that a sugar pill or placebo. The second consultant who is called in refers to a clinician trained in our viewpoint and protocol. The clinician sees the problem emanating from within the individual. In our allegory the new consultant offers the solution we suggest, which is aimed at rehabilitating the chronically contracted posture of the tissues in the pelvic floor as well as teaching the individual to cease the habitual and chronic pelvic tensing.

In our allegory, we make the point that 'the world' has lost communication with the pelvis. Most of our patients tend to be out of touch with what is going on in their pelvis. We offer a method to open communication with the pelvis to help bring about a healing of the sore and irritated pelvic tissues.

Healing pelvic muscles by changing bad habits

If chronic tension results in an irritation of selective contents of the pelvic floor that gives rise to pain, then anything one does to reduce or eliminate the tension has the potential of eliminating the pain. *The restoration of the contracted tissues to a normal state of flexibility and relaxation has to be done repetitively.*

It is the repetitive application of our methods that gives the pelvic muscles a chance to return to their normal state. In later chapters, we introduce the methods used to accomplish this called *Paradoxical Relaxation and Myofascial/Trigger Point Release. Paradoxical Relaxation*, discussed in depth in this book, trains the patient to break the habit of chronically tensing the pelvic muscles. *Myofascial/Trigger Point Release* makes it possible for the pelvic muscles to adequately relax through the aid of a therapist who literally lengthens the constricted pelvic tissue.

We tell our patients to expect ups and down, and not to celebrate when symptoms reduce, or to despair when they flare-up. This is easy to say and not so easy to do when you are anxious and in pain.

There are important reasons why chronic pelvic pain syndromes are misunderstood and why progress is slow. One reason is that the pelvic muscles are almost always active in the service of the normal functions in life. The pelvic muscles need a rest from their chronic contraction.

There are two factors that make this difficult. The first is that you can't simply rest the pelvic muscles for any extended period. They are needed to allow you to stand up, to hold in urine, to walk, to lift—to do the things that allow you to be able to function normally. It is a delicate juggling act to deal with the need for rest and healing of this vital part of the body on the one hand and the demand on the pelvic muscles to do the work required to function in life.

The other factor that operates against the healing of the pelvic floor is the conditioned tendency to focus tension in it when under stress. This is usually a deeply ingrained tendency, especially when this focus of tension has been practiced many times without awareness. Modifying this habit so that contracting the pelvic muscles under stress is *not* the default mode is no small enterprise. Changing this habit is the focus of the method of *Paradoxical Relaxation.*

In our allegory, we show that while the intervention of the second consultant began helping the situation, the situation did not immediately go back to normal. The process of healing takes time, especially inside an active pelvic floor.

Reassurance and emotional support helps pelvic pain syndrome

Harry Miller, M.D. from the Department of Urology at George Washington University reported on his treatment of men who had prostatitis. Dr. Miller offered stress management therapy. He gave them very simple and kindly advice not unlike that of a grandmother to her grandson. Miller's approach reinforced the idea to his patients that there was a relationship between how they managed the stress in their life and their symptoms. In doing so he helped most of his patients reduce their symptoms.

Dr. Miller's work focused on the person and not the prostate. He addressed the social and psychological context in which pelvic pain occurs. Similarly, the approach discussed in this book insists that chronic pelvic pain syndromes are a problem of the person which includes, but is not limited to, a sore part of the person's body.

What seems obvious may not be the problem: the source of the disorder in interstitial cystitis may not simply be the bladder

The focus of the problem in interstitial cystitis (IC) may not be limited to the bladder, but found in the muscles of the pelvic floor. Treatment protocols in traditional medicine have focused exclusively on the bladder.

Some compelling evidence throws doubt on this view that the bladder is the essential problem in IC. One study showed that when the pelvic muscles of patients with IC were palpated, the pelvic muscles appeared to be the source of the pain. The bladder was rarely found to be painful when touched. In a Finnish study, 25 of 31 women who were diagnosed with IC reported pain in the pelvic muscles and not in the bladder when the bladder and the pelvic floor were palpated.

Perhaps even more compelling is the experience we had with a patient whose level of pain with IC prompted a physician to remove the bladder. The bladder removal did not reduce the pain. Unfortunately this is not the only patient whose bladder was removed and whose pain persisted.

We are suggesting that the source of the problem with IC may not be the bladder. Instead, the source may be the nerves, muscles, and blood vessels in the pelvic floor connecting to the bladder.

Our multidisciplinary treatment protocol

Our multidisciplinary treatment team for the Stanford protocol is comprised of a urologist, a psychologist, and a physical therapist. The urologist does the initial diagnosis and makes sure that the condition is appropriate for our protocol. His or her work involves an examination of the patient, the administration of various medical tests, and interpretation of the results. It is the physician's findings that rule out serious illness as a factor in the patient's symptoms. He examines and maps out the pelvic floor for trigger points and areas of restriction. Then either he or a physical therapist administers the intrapelvic *Myofascial/Trigger Point Release.*

The psychologist's primary role in the treatment team is to train the patient in *Paradoxical Relaxation* for the purpose of profoundly relaxing the pelvic floor and modifying the habit of focusing tension in the pelvic floor under stress. The psychologist on our team teaches a method to help the patient stop the catastrophic and negative thinking associated with the condition of pelvic pain and dysfunction. This method requires regular practice as the negative thinking arises during the course of a day. The method is simple and easily learned and applied.

To facilitate continued *Myofascial/Trigger Point Release* therapy in the home setting, whenever possible, the willing spouse or partner is taught the method. The physical therapist teaches the patient to self administer the internal myofascial release and gives instructions for a home program of stretches, not unlike a home yoga program, except that these stretches are oriented toward the rehabilitation of the chronically tensed pelvic muscles.

Members of these different disciplines work well together as they hold the same cross-disciplinary understanding of the problem being treated and collaborate with each other on treatment.

The treatment is most likely to help when you reduce the stress in your life

John B., a 38 year-old small business owner, came to see us with pelvic pain and urinary dysfunction. Upon examining him, we determined that in fact, he had no problems of an organic nature. He had trigger points inside his pelvic floor that when palpated exactly recreated his symptoms.

Under normal circumstances, John was someone we would be very optimistic about being able to help but it became clear he was not. He owned a car repair facility where he employed 45 people, and his business consumed his days from 6 in the morning until 9 at night. His wife was unhappy because of his absence from their relationship. His children had behavioral and academic problems at school. He was also involved in a lawsuit with his brother-in-law with whom he had owned a previous business. He was in the middle of a major renovation of his house that left both he and his wife sleeping on a mattress on the floor.

John had no time for himself, let alone the time to do physical therapy and daily relaxation to relax his pelvic floor. Under these circumstances, the program we offered would have been ineffective because he would not be able to do it properly in the face of the demands and stress calling for his attention. Only when John himself decided that his life would have to change would our treatment have a chance to help him resolve his pelvic pain.

Effective treatment requires adherence to the complete program

Patients who seem to get the best results from our treatment are those who are clearly committed to earnestly practicing our approach. Usually these patients have suffered for a long time and have seen numerous doctors and explored many avenues. These patients often assume the attitude of "I will do whatever it takes to get better" and have no problem following the protocol. We tend to discourage patients who are skittish or unsure about doing our treatment. These are usually patients whose level of pain and dysfunction is minimal and who have been suffering for a short period of time.

Chronic pelvic pain as a functional disorder

Prostatitis and other chronic pelvic pain syndromes can be understood as 'functional disorders.' This viewpoint is most clearly expressed by Dr. Jeanette Potts, a physician and researcher at the Cleveland Clinic, who has maintained that nonbacterial prostatitis and chronic pelvic pain syndromes are functional disorders. Pelvic pain syndromes are defined by the fact that these conditions show no glaring physical abnormalities to account for the pain and suffering they cause. They are defined as a problem in function, not in structure. In other words, the structures within the pelvic floor of those with chronic pelvic pain syndromes tend to have healthy structures that display a disturbance in function. Hence they are a functional disorder.

Having a functional disorder does not mean it is all in your head

We do not dismiss functional disorders as any less real than a broken bone. More than a few patients have told us that they have seen doctors who have told them that there is nothing wrong and that they should either live with their condition or go to a psychiatrist. This is naturally disturbing to a patient who is faced with his doctor telling him that his pain and dysfunction are somehow not real or untreatable.

People with functional disorders often have more than one

In our practice, we have noticed that there is a high incidence of irritable bowel syndrome in patients who also have pelvic pain. Given the proximity of the colon and the pelvis, it makes sense that both could be the result of a chronic abdominal/pelvic tension. While gastroenterology and urology make a distinction between the urogenital system and gastrointestinal tract, the body doesn't necessarily make any such distinctions or recognize any such boundaries.

The concepts of threshold, pelvic pain, and functional disorders

When first facing pelvic pain, one faces what seems to be a monolithic, undifferentiated curtain of pain and distress that feels incomprehensible and overwhelming. Patients usually feel helpless in the face of pelvic pain because they know little or nothing about what they can do about their condition. Therefore, the concept of a threshold, and proximity to the threshold, is often a useful idea to patients so that a perspective can be gained on one's progress.

We assess the effectiveness of our treatment by looking at the presence, intensity, and frequency of symptoms. Consider the following scheme. The symptom threshold is the point your pelvic tension and irritability reaches in order to produce pain and dysfunction. You can locate your proximity to the threshold, above which you are symptomatic and below which you are not. When patients are able to see their symptoms from the viewpoint of their proximity to the symptom threshold, they can gauge their progress and relieve their sense of helplessness and confusion when their symptoms wax and wane.

One's proximity to the symptom threshold

#4   Chronically symptomatic

#3   Symptoms wax and wane

SYMPTOM THRESHOLD

#2   No symptoms when slightly below
     threshold; can become symptomatic at the
     slightest stress

#1   No symptoms

In the threshold schema, the person who is located in position #1 is well below the threshold, displays no symptoms, and can tolerate a great amount of tension in the pelvic floor without becoming symptomatic. Even when this person's pelvic tension goes over the threshold the pelvic tissue is not irritated, and the pelvic floor muscles are flexible and immediately drop below the threshold after the individual has stopped tensing. The person in this position has a normal, healthy pelvis.

The person situated in position #2 represents someone who likely will have pelvic pain but on an intermittent basis. It does not take great increases in pelvic tension to throw this person's tension level above the threshold where he or she will become symptomatic. The person at position #2, generally speaking, has a reduced level of flexibility in the pelvic floor and often does not relax as easily as someone in position #1 once the muscles are tensed over the level of the threshold.

People with pelvic pain who are in position #2 are often bewildered at what brings on their symptoms. They conclude that there was nothing much that seemed to be associated with the onset of symptoms, and that the pain is random. Our explanation is that when someone is slightly below the threshold what a non-event is for a normal person is often stressful enough to throw a #2 over the threshold and into symptoms.

At position #3 is the individual who has mild but persistent symptoms that wax and wane. This is the person who is 'surfing' the threshold. Symptoms associated with #3, while seeming to be almost always present, occasionally drop below threshold only to come back inexplicably. The person at position #3 usually experiences chronic but more or less tolerable pain and dysfunction.

At position #4 is the individual who has chronic and intractable pelvic pain and/or dysfunction. He or she doesn't drop below the symptom threshold. When asked to describe the frequency and severity of symptoms, this person will report that the symptoms are always present, 24 hours a day, seven days a week, and that the symptoms strongly impact his or her life. Our treatment aims to lower baseline pelvic tension and irritability of individuals in positions #2, #3, and #4 to that of the position #1.

Anxiety increases your symptoms

Most of the patients we see with chronic pelvic pain syndromes have what we have referred to earlier in this chapter as trigger points in their pelvic muscles. The way we determine the existence of trigger points is discussed in the section on *Myofascial/Trigger Point Release*. To reiterate, a trigger point is a taut band within a muscle that is painful either spontaneously or when touched and which creates pain at the site palpated or refers pain to a site remote from it. Trigger points are exquisitely sensitive and it is not uncommon for the patient to jump when the trigger point is pressed. We determine the presence of a trigger point through a digital/rectal or digital/vaginal examination. The doctor inserts a finger inside the rectum or vagina and presses on the muscles to assess the tissue and to find trigger points.

A 1994 study sheds much light on the relationship between trigger points and stress. McNulty, Gevertz, Hubbard, and Berkoff inserted a needle electrode directly into a trigger point and monitored its electrical activity with a machine called an electromyograph. It appears that the higher the electrical activity in a trigger point, the higher the level of pain.

Patients were given the stressful task of doing mental arithmetic. The scientists wanted to determine what the effects of stress were on the trigger points being monitored and the differences, if any, between the responses of the trigger points and the responses of the adjacent non-sensitive tissue without trigger points. Results indicated that the electrical activity of the trigger points increased during this stressful activity while the adjacent, non-trigger point tissue remained electrically unresponsive.

These findings are remarkable. They suggest that in some way the nervous system that is connected to the stress of emotional activity and arousal is selectively connected to trigger points and not to non-trigger point tissue. Understanding this, it is easy to understand why patients with pelvic pain and dysfunction routinely report that their symptoms are aggravated by stress.

Anxiety, anger, fear and sorrow, which are expressions of nervous system arousal, can cause increased pain in areas that have trigger points. Furthermore, your fearful attitude toward your body and symptoms can stress you. If you are aware of pain every day during urination or sexual activity, and you feel anxious each time you are aware of your pain, it is clearly very important to shift your thoughts and attitude about your symptoms.

Plato taught that we need to be kind to each other because each of us is engaged in a mighty struggle in our lives. Compassion for the most difficult of people comes from understanding their struggle. Like letting go of anger and fear toward difficult people, letting go of fear and anxiety toward a painful rectum and genitals is simply an expression of your understanding and compassion for your own struggle. Discovering compassion toward oneself and one's body is part of our protocol. As patients understand the language of the pelvic floor and their struggle with their habit of chronically tightening it, their attitude can change from fear to compassion and understanding.

What is the role of inflammation?

As one views the maladies and aberrations that occur in the human body to create suffering—particularly from pain—the evidence for inflammatory conditions underlying a great preponderance of these disorders is plentiful: coronary artery disease, arthritis, inflammatory bowel disease, multiple neurologic disorders, diabetes, infectious diseases, etc., and the list goes on and on. We have no reason to think that chronic pelvic pain disorders may not also be an inflammatory condition. However, the problem is an almost total lack of any convincing evidence that an inflammatory condition is responsible for pelvic pain. Are trigger points inflamed? The answer is unknown.

A few things are known and others strongly believed. There is a large literature that shows that inflammation produces anxiety. But there is also significant evidence that anxiety is a pro-inflammatory state and anxiety may worsen inflammatory conditions and even cancer deterioration. Whether it is surgery, infection, arthritis, cancer, coronary disease or bowel disease, stress and distress can worsen inflammation. Stress is well known to delay wound healing. For example, if you are among those who score in the top one-third of anxiety behavior, you will take four times as long to heal a duodenal ulcer. The association between anxiety and inflammation, in our view, is one of the reasons that makes it imperative to bring ongoing anxiety, so frequently connected to pelvic pain and dysfunction, under control.

Some inflammatory conditions of the body are obviously harmful to us. Parts of our body become the collateral damage from the war that the body wages when anything remotely threatening to our survival becomes involved. Certain kinds of defense cells found in the inflammatory response may secrete noxious and toxic biochemicals that cause pain. Inflammation almost always overshoots the mark and then we have to suffer from it. The scientific evidence would suggest that reduction of stress can promote healing and reduce the inflammatory response.

More discussion concerning the role of inflammation associated with the chronic pelvic pain syndromes can be found in Chapter 9. Suffice it to say that we applaud the efforts of physicians and scientists to uncover the pathologic mechanisms whereby chronic pelvic pain is created. Our efforts are immediately directed to providing a new ways of thinking about the problem of pelvic pain, confronting it with readily available tools that are not additionally harmful to the body, and accepting the generous gift of being able to make a difference in the daily ravages of this terrible pain condition.

Chronic tension leads to anxiety and pain

Chronic pelvic pain has been resistant to effective treatment because of what we call the *tension, anxiety, pain cycle*. This is a cycle in which chronic tension has shortened the muscles in the pelvic floor and created an environment in which the pelvic floor can be said to be functioning like a clenched fist. This leads to pain and dysfunction. The pain is a signal of alarm to which the body responds with protective bracing and a heightened state of arousal or anxiety. Anxiety always produces increased tension, which then produces more pain, which then produces more anxiety.

The Tension-Anxiety-Pain Cycle

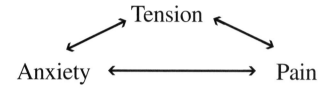

The tension, anxiety and pain cycle is the heart of the problem of most chronic pelvic pain syndromes we treat. Once the pelvis becomes sore, painful and the normal functions are disturbed in some way, the sore and painful pelvis becomes hyper-sensitive to anxiety. Anxiety tightens in preparation for fight or flight. This tightening of the pelvic floor and surrounding musculature tends to be reflexive and usually happens out of a person's awareness. Some level of anxiety is what almost all patients with chronic pelvic pain syndromes live with day in and day out. Anxiety can regularly exacerbate the condition fed by the patients catastrophic thinking, the isolation of sharing one's feelings with very few, and a medical establishment that can't help.

In the presence of anxiety, the sore pelvis can't fully relax. This relaxation is necessary for the healing of the sore pelvic tissue. Added to an individual's anxiety is the puzzlement of the doctors whom the individual sees for this problem. The doctor is often frustrated about his inability to help the problem and is not infrequently worried that perhaps he has missed something. Doctors are problem solvers. Certain doctors, particularly, do not respond well to their helplessness to solve the problem of pelvic pain. Any anxiety, uncertainty or helplessness of the doctor is almost always communicated to the patient–a communication whose impact is profound. Who wouldn't be troubled by chronic pelvic pain and dysfunction in which your doctor couldn't help you?

Pelvic pain is hugely affected and perpetuated by anxiety. This is why the placebo effect is so great in these conditions because they temporarily reduce the anxiety that tends to fuel the condition. This is also why many people have a reduction in symptoms after they read this book. Finally something makes sense about what is going on and offers some intuitively viable solution.

We often see patients in pain who are very emotionally upset about their pain on an ongoing basis. Their hands are often cold and clammy; they are agitated and can't seem to sit still. These patients are caught in the active grip of *the tension-anxiety-pain cycle.*

The difficulty of intervening effectively on behalf of these patients is illustrated in the children's jump rope game called "double Dutch." In this game, two children facing each other, turn two ropes, one clockwise, and the other counter-clockwise, as one child jumps both of the ropes.

The difficulty in double Dutch is found in entering through both swinging ropes into the jumping space. Children who successfully "jump double Dutch" are able to watch the two ropes as they follow closely one after another and to determine the split second when there is a space through which they can enter. Even for an athletic and bright child, double Dutch is a challenge. Similarly, the events that occur in the *tension-anxiety-pain cycle* follow so closely one after the other, that we could call this "triple Dutch." Entering into these events to stop the cycle is not a small challenge.

A gentle approach to break the tension-anxiety-pain cycle

We intervene in this cycle in all three of its aspects. *Paradoxical Relaxation* lowers pelvic tension and anxiety by lowering autonomic nervous system arousal in general, and habitual pelvic tension, in particular. *Myofascial/Trigger Point Release* deactivates trigger point pain, lengthens chronically contracted muscles, and makes the pelvic muscles more capable of relaxation. We have found that an effective way of beginning therapy, when someone is caught in the grips of the *tension-anxiety-pain cycle*, is to start treatment gradually. If the patient cannot tolerate any pressure inside the rectum or vagina, we begin the physical part of our treatment by simply inserting a finger with no pressure anywhere. If they cannot tolerate the insertion of the finger, we hold the finger gently, touching the opening of the rectum or vagina without moving at all. In backing up and reducing the intensity of the treatment to a tolerable level, we find a baseline from which to begin.

John J., a patient from Minneapolis, could not tolerate any pressure inside his pelvic floor. When we instructed his wife in the *Myofascial/ Trigger Point Release,* we told her to simply insert her finger inside his rectum and not to press anywhere. She did this on a daily basis for a week, and with our instruction, she began slightly pressing on a trigger point. Gradually, as her husband could tolerate more, she increased the pressure. After a few months, he was able to tolerate the pressure that we are usually able to exert at the beginning of treatment with most other patients.

Similarly, John J. was not able to lie down and do the first lesson in the relaxation training for more than three minutes. We instructed him to do *Paradoxical Relaxation* for two minutes each day, which he did for a week or so. Following this, we increased the relaxation time gradually until he reported actually relaxing for over a period of half an hour.

In summary, it is when you can find a method to rehabilitate the chronically tensed and shortened muscles, restore their original length and flexibility, and change the habit of continually squeezing them and the nerves, blood vessels and structures they contain that a substantial number of patients with previously untreatable pelvic pain can experience a marked improvement or complete abatement of symptoms.

Our understanding is a significant departure from the conventional view of prostatitis and chronic pelvic pain syndromes. We see pelvic pain as often being a physical expression of the way a person copes with life. We propose that *pelvic pain is the result of a neuromuscular state perpetuated by anxiety and chronic bracing and not the result of a foreign organism in the prostate gland or an autoimmune disorder. When certain predisposed individuals focus tension in the pelvic muscles*, this chronic tension over time, creates an inhospitable environment in the pelvic floor that gives rise to tension, anxiety, and pain. *Once the cycle of tension, anxiety, and pain is set into motion, it takes on a life of its own. Our treatment aims to restore the capacity of the pelvic tissue to relax, to perform its normal functions, and to return to a pain-free and dysfunction-free state.* This rehabilitative protocol consists of the simultaneous use of *Paradoxical Relaxation* and *Myofascial/Trigger Point Release.*

CHAPTER 4

THE STANFORD PROTOCOL: PARADOXICAL RELAXATION AND MYOFASCIAL/TRIGGER POINT RELEASE

Introduction to the methodology

- *Paradoxical Relaxation* teaches the skill of profoundly relaxing the muscles of the pelvis and modifying the habit of focusing tension in the pelvic floor under stress. The skill is developed by repetitive practice of the proper technique.

- *Myofascial/Trigger Point Release* is a manual technique of deactivating pain referring trigger points, stretching, loosening, and lengthening the contracted tissue inside and outside the pelvic floor, thereby enabling it to relax. The technique focuses on trigger points and areas of spasm and constriction.

Once a patient has been diagnosed and considered appropriate for our treatment, he or she begins combined therapy with *Paradoxical Relaxation* and intrapelvic *Myofascial/Trigger Point Release*. *Paradoxical Relaxation* aims to relax the grip of pelvic tension that does not allow the pelvis to relax and heal its chronic state of hyperirritability. Furthermore its aim is to modify the long-standing habit of focusing tension in the pelvic muscles. Our goal is to help a patient become skilled in deeply relaxing the pelvic muscles at will.

The *Myofascial/Trigger Point Release* aims to free the muscles in and around the pelvis of active trigger points and to restore the muscles of the pelvic floor to a flexible and lengthened state. This is done by performing a specialized type of internal and external therapy that deactivates painful trigger points and mobilizes the soft tissue of the pelvic floor. In this aspect of treatment, a therapist is in direct digital contact with the physical sites of the pain and constriction. The purpose of this intervention is to slowly stretch the constricted pelvic tissue to a normal length and level of flexibility.

It is our view that *when Paradoxical Relaxation or Myofascial/Trigger Point Release is done in the absence of the other, the potential reduction or elimination of symptoms is substantially reduced.*

Who is appropriate for the methodology?

We determine that someone is an appropriate candidate for our treatment after a thorough diagnostic evaluation. This evaluation is necessary to rule out organic conditions that might be mimicking the symptoms of the conditions we treat. It is essential that we know what we are treating.

The recommended treatment is most effective when patients are not currently using medications. This is not always possible. Many patients have been given antibiotics, alpha blockers, muscle relaxants and pain killers, and have grown reliant upon them. We recommend that whenever possible, and under medical supervision, the patient weans off of these medications before starting treatment. This isn't absolutely essential to begin treatment but advised when possible.

We have had our best results when we have been able to find trigger points internally and/or externally that tend to recreate a patient's symptoms. Determining this is a skill in which few physicians or physical therapists have experience. Determining whether or not someone has trigger points that recreate symptoms usually requires our evaluation. In our chapter on *Myofascial / Trigger Point Release* in this book, we describe and show illustrations of the most common trigger points related to pelvic pain.

Some individuals have written us to ask if an unremarkable biofeedback reading rules them out for our protocol. In another section of this book we have indicated *that a pelvic floor biofeedback reading is an unreliable criterion for determining the appropriateness of our protocol. In other words, a rectal or vaginal biofeedback sensor that indicates a normal amount of tension is not a reason to rule out the appropriateness of our protocol. Pelvic floor electromyographic evaluation of the anal sphincter or the opening of the vagina is one of those medical tests in which a positive finding may be significant and point toward the proper therapy, whereas a negative result may not prove anything.*

We believe that the use of narcotic pain medicines tends to lower a person's pain threshold and often leads to habituation or addiction. There are a few patients we have helped who began treatment while taking narcotic medications, and have been able to wean themselves of these medications during the course of treatment.

A strong motivation to do our rigorous protocol that often takes 1-1/2 hours per day for the first number of months is essential to the success of our treatment. If someone is not adequately motivated, it is unlikely that the person will be a good candidate for our work.

Assessing the Symptoms of Our Patients

Below are the forms we use to evaluate people's symptoms before treatment begins. They are also filled out at each visit. These scores are relative for each person and do allow us to compare the scores over time and to assess a patient's progress. The form is divided into sections on pelvic pain, urinary dysfunction, and sexual difficulties. The *Pelvic Pain Symptom Score* questionnaire used with our Stanford protocol is a modification of a survey developed by Dr. John Krieger, University of Washington, and as well, incorporates survey questions from the American Urological Association.

Pelvic Pain Symptom Score Form (Male)

Name_____ Date_____

Over the past month or so, including today, how much were you bothered by:

	Not at all		Moderate		Extreme
Pain in the lower back	0	1	2	3	4
Pain in the lower abdomen	0	1	2	3	4
Pain during urination	0	1	2	3	4
Pain with bowel movements	0	1	2	3	4
Pain in rectum	0	1	2	3	4
Pain in the prostate gland	0	1	2	3	4
Pain in the testicles	0	1	2	3	4
Pain in the penis	0	1	2	3	4

Number of days experienced pain in the last month _____ days
How bad is the pain on average now? 0_____10
                                                    no pain   worst pain

Total Pain Score_____

Difficulty postponing urination, hard to hold it (urgency)	0	1	2	3	4
Need to urinate again less than 2 hours after urinating (frequency)	0	1	2	3	4

Number of times urinating at night	0	1	2	3	4
Bladder does not feel completely empty after urinating	0	1	2	3	4
Stopping and starting several times while urinating (intermittency)	0	1	2	3	4
Weak urinary stream	0	1	2	3	4
Having to push or strain to begin urination	0	1	2	3	4

Total Urinary Score _____

Lack of interest in sexual activity	0	1	2	3	4
Difficulty getting an erection	0	1	2	3	4
Difficulty maintaining an erection	0	1	2	3	4
Difficulty reaching an ejaculation	0	1	2	3	4
Pain with ejaculation	0	1	2	3	4
Pain or discomfort after ejaculation	0	1	2	3	4

Total Sexual Score _____

In addition, men also fill out the National Institutes of Health-Chronic Prostatitis Symptom Index as a comparison tool.

Pelvic Pain Symptom Score Form (Female)

Name_____ Date_____

Over the past month or so, including today, how much were you bothered by:

	Not at all		Moderate		Extreme
Pain in the lower back	0	1	2	3	4
Pain in the lower abdomen	0	1	2	3	4
Pain during urination	0	1	2	3	4
Pain with bowel movements	0	1	2	3	4
Pain in rectum	0	1	2	3	4
Pain in the urethra	0	1	2	3	4
Pain in the vagina	0	1	2	3	4
Pain with menstrual period	0	1	2	3	4
Pain with intercourse	0	1	2	3	4

Number of days experienced pain in the last month _____ days

How bad is the pain on average now? 0_____10

                                no pain   worst pain

Total Pain Score_____

Urinary urgency/frequency	0	1	2	3	4
Number of times urinating at night	0	1	2	3	4
Difficulty emptying the bladder	0	1	2	3	4

Total Urinary Score_____

An overview of what happens in treatment:
the six-day intensive clinic for the Stanford Protocol

Paradoxical Relaxation originally was taught during office consultations. Patients were given an audiocassette course in *Paradoxical Relaxation* to be used daily at home. Follow-up was provided by regular consultations at Stanford or by telephone or internet consultations for those who lived at a distance.

The intrapelvic *Myofascial/Trigger Point Release* was originally performed over a number of months in a series of office visits. The typical course of treatment involved ten to forty individual sessions, each lasting between thirty to sixty minutes. Our protocol usually began with two or three physical therapy sessions per week, tapering down as the rehabilitation of the pelvic floor occurred.

While we sometimes continue to treat patients by seeing them in the office on a weekly basis, we have discovered that the best way to do our protocol is in the form of a six-day intensive clinic which we do monthly. These are intensive clinics in which patients immerse themselves in the protocol. Patients learn the relaxation protocol more easily and more thoroughly, having many hours to experience the method, deal with the difficulties that normally arise and have their questions cleared up. Absence from their regular life and routine provides an opportunity for the nervous system to significantly quiet down. We have seen symptoms reduce more quickly among certain patients during the clinics than in the one-session per week format.

The physical therapist has an opportunity to see the patient daily, to follow up on what transpired in the session the day earlier, and to go into a depth of exploration of the pelvic floor that is often not possible in a weekly single visit. Most important, we have the luxury of time to teach the self-treatment protocol and make sure patients have a clear understanding and competence in this protocol.

When someone has a willing partner, we teach the partner how to perform the *Myofascial/Trigger Point Release*. This involvement of the partner usually shortens the number of visits to the physical therapist or physician.

We have developed a myofascial/trigger point wand for self-administered myofascial/trigger point treatment. While we are still evaluating the efficacy of this wand, it has helped a group of patients to be able to reach and release certain internal trigger points. It is still in an experimental stage; however we now can prescribe it to selected patients. Use of this wand at home is done with careful instruction and supervision.

Our Purpose is to Make A Pain-Free State the Normal State

Tissue memory: nerves, muscles, and blood vessels adapt to their situation

Researchers in the area of pain have tried to understand why pain becomes chronic even in the absence of any objective physical findings. The explanation that is emerging revolves around the idea that the tissues themselves have memory and can 'remember' and recreate the pain even when the original source of it has gone away.

We see the evidence of tissue memory in our work with pelvic pain and dysfunction. Earlier we discussed some patients with pain and dysfunction from interstitial cystitis who opted for surgery to have their bladders removed. Choosing such a radical approach was based on the idea that if the source of the pain was removed, which presumably was the bladder, the pain would be gone. Unfortunately, after surgery, the pain remained unabated in these patients.

From the point of view of tissue memory, we might say that the bladder originally may have been the source of the pain. The nerves, muscles, and blood vessels that connected to the bladder may have "remembered" the pain circuits even when the bladder was removed. The removal of the bladder did not address the tissue memory that participated in and enabled the pain in the first place.

Adapting to chronic pain

No one with pelvic pain and dysfunction says that their symptoms feel comfortable or normal. However, it may be that your body has adapted to your pain and dysfunction as a normal state. In other words, your pelvic pain and dysfunction at a certain level may become 'home' and a place of stability.

It is often the case that patients will experience significant relief from symptoms after both *Paradoxical Relaxation* and *Myofascial/Trigger Point Release.* This relief is often brief, with symptoms re-emerging after hours or days. In our view, the 'normal' setting was shifted from one of pain to one of less or no pain. This setting needs to be reestablished as 'normal' by repeating treatment over and over again. *One purpose of Myofascial/Trigger Point Release and Paradoxical Relaxation is to retrain the nerves, muscles, and blood vessels so that freedom from pain and dysfunction feels like home.*

An example: getting used to not stuttering

In 1971 Dr. Martin Schwartz, professor of speech science, department of surgery at New York University, noted spasms of the vocal cords in a patient who stuttered during blocked efforts at speaking. When she was able to speak again, her vocal cords slightly relaxed, enough for air to pass through and vibrate them. This insight led him to a new treatment for stuttering that allowed most stutterers using his method to stop stuttering within a few minutes. Success was achieved by learning a simple respiratory maneuver that prevented the vocal cords from locking immediately prior to speaking.

The biggest challenge to stopping stuttering, Schwartz reported, was changing the stutterer's unconscious resistance to not stuttering. For stutterers, stuttering is known territory. Though uncomfortable and dysfunctional, stuttering and everything associated with it is familiar and known. As one stutterer reported to Dr. Schwartz, "I don't stutter now, but my problem is no knowing how to talk to people."

A dysfunctional state can become home. Fluent speech, to the unconscious mind and highly practiced conditioning of the stutterer, can feel destabilizing and threatening.

Schwarz states "Give them effective techniques, have them practice the techniques regularly so they become semi-automatic and then take them through a hierarchy of situations graded with respect to stress, moving from initially low stress to increasingly greater degrees of stress." The Schwartz method enables stutterers to overcome their anticipatory fear that drove their stuttering. It is a method that enables many stutterers to make fluency feel like "home."

Paradoxical Relaxation and the Profound Relaxation of the Pelvic Floor

The aim of Paradoxical Relaxation

People with chronic pelvic pain have a tendency to focus tension in the pelvic floor under stress. Over time this focus of tension shortens the pelvic muscles and makes an inhospitable environment for the muscles, nerves, tissues, and structures involved in the pelvic floor. This inhospitable environment contributes to the symptoms we normally associate with chronic pelvic pain.

The shortened state of the muscles inside the pelvic floor does not allow for normal relaxation and flexibility of the tissue. *Myofascial/*

Trigger Point Release is necessary to deactivate the pain-referring trigger points and to loosen the constricted muscles and make it possible for them to relax. The impediment to this relaxation, however, is the often deeply ingrained habit of tensing the pelvic muscles under stress.

The aim of *Paradoxical Relaxation*, therefore, is to change the habit of automatically tensing in the pelvic floor. Furthermore, the relaxation of the pelvic muscles helps to create the essential healing environment necessary for the irritated nerves, tissues, and structures of the pelvic floor. The repetitive relaxation of the pelvic floor allows for the regeneration of tissue, proper oxygenation, nutrition, and waste management of the tissues. Regularly quieting of the autonomic nervous system helps the pelvic muscles get used to no pain or dysfunction as the normal state.

It is not obvious how to begin to teach someone to relax when there is pain. Without any training, people in pain clearly have difficulty relaxing. They remain tense as the body tries to guard itself against the pain. This is understandable, even natural, but in the long run, it is not helpful. *The key to relaxing a painful and contracted pelvic floor is to restore the contracted pelvic tissue to a state so that it has the capacity to relax using Paradoxical Relaxation described here.*

When you are relaxing while you are in pain your goal at first is to subtract tension and discomfort rather than aiming to entirely eliminate it. In this section we will discuss the origins of *Paradoxical Relaxation* and the details of its technique.

Origins of Paradoxical Relaxation: the work of Edmund Jacobson

The foundation of *Paradoxical Relaxation* began almost eighty years ago with the work of Dr. Edmund Jacobson and his method of *Progressive Relaxation*. *Progressive Relaxation* has been the father of most relaxation methods used in western medicine and has been used in one form or another throughout most of the twentieth century. Over the years, many research studies have been done on the effect of *Progressive Relaxation* on conditions varying from constipation to ringing in the ears. Jacobson's method has stood the test of time.

The background in which Jacobson's work developed

Jacobson was born in 1888 to a middle class family in Chicago. A brilliant student, he graduated from Northwestern University in two years. At the age of 18 he attended Harvard University where he was the youngest to receive a Ph.D. in psychology at that time. He taught physiology at the University of Chicago and later went to Rush Medical College where he received a degree as a Doctor of Medicine.

Jacobson related that when he was eight years old, a fire broke out at an apartment house owned by his parents in turn of the century Chicago. Tragically, a close friend of his parents was killed in the blaze and his parents became distraught and hysterical over this shocking loss.

The level of his parents' upset deeply disturbed the young Jacobson. He reported later in his life that at the time of the fire, he vowed never to get upset the way his parents had gotten upset. This desire to remain calm and relaxed stayed with him through adolescence.

Later, when dealing with his insomnia as an undergraduate at Harvard, he began to experiment with his own methods of relaxation. As he developed a technique that allowed him to go to sleep, he chose to write his Ph.D. dissertation on an experiment showing that tense subjects responded acutely to a stressor (two metal bars clanging), while subjects trained in relaxation hardly reacted at all.

Jacobson was the master of his method. A newspaper reporter who interviewed Jacobson toward the end of his life wrote that she acutely felt the level of her own nervousness through the mirror of being around such a profoundly calm man. It was his ability to relax deeply and reduce his metabolic requirements for oxygen that allowed him to stay underwater for several minutes.

When he demonstrated his relaxation method in front of students, he was able to relax so deeply in a minute or two that he looked like a corpse because the only muscles that had any appreciable tension were the muscles required for the functioning of his heart and for respiration. Perhaps the greatest demonstration of his mastery of relaxation was his long life of 95 years especially in light of the fact that both his parents had died at relatively young ages.

Jacobson's life was devoted to applying the principles he developed to the treatment of many psychosomatic disorders. In 1924 he treated women with *globus hystericus*, a condition in which the patient feels that there is something stuck in the throat. Jacobson documented the narrowing of the esophagus in this condition by capturing images of the esophagus with a fluoroscope. He then trained these patients in *Progressive Relaxation* and fluoroscoped the esophagus after the relaxation training. Not only were the subjective symptoms resolved, but the fluoroscopic images verified a widening of the constricted portions of the esophagus.

For the next 60 years, the conditions Jacobson successfully treated included hypertension, spastic esophagus, spastic colon, headache, functional cardiac disorders like heart palpitation and arrhythmia, as well as the gamut of psychological disorders including anxiety disorders, depression, and mania. He documented the success of his treatment in the many studies he published. What is perhaps more remarkable is that Jacobson proposed the link between stress and illness many decades before it became fashionable. It is also remarkable that he actually treated patients and conducted scientific research on the subject at a time where there was very little interest and awareness on the relationship between body and mind.

In the mid-1940s Jacobson wanted to develop a machine that would be able to independently verify the efficacy of his method. There were no reliable independent findings that could indicate whether someone was relaxed or whether there was any change in their level of relaxation as the result of Jacobson's intervention.

In conjunction with Bell Telephone Laboratories he developed the first *electromyograph*, an instrument able to detect electrical activity in muscles with a sensitivity of up to one millionth of a volt. With this machine the formerly undetectable physiologic effects could be easily and scientifically demonstrated. The *electromyograph* could *objectively verify* whether someone was tense or relaxed and the extent to which *Progressive Relaxation* had an effect.

Although the *electromyograph* formed the basis of the first biofeedback machine, Jacobson was never interested in incorporating the technological wonder he created as a tool in the clinical setting. He took a position that one could not learn to relax while looking at a meter or listening to a tone. He felt that the very act of looking or listening was tension producing and interfered with dropping into the profound states of relaxation for which he was aiming.

Progressive Relaxation is best known for its instruction to contract and relax muscles at the beginning of relaxation. In fact, many practitioners who have not understood *Progressive Relaxation* have thought that it simply involves voluntarily tightening and then relaxing muscles as a way of promoting relaxation in the muscles. This is a fundamental misunderstanding.

Jacobson was clear that his instruction to tense and then relax a muscle was intended to only highlight tension so that the patient could consciously recognize how it felt. *The ability to recognize subtle degrees of tension is a master skill in Progressive Relaxation.* The most difficult patients to treat are those who report that they feel very little or no tension, even though they have obvious tension by objective measures.

The contract/relax instruction in large part was meant to help patients who were out of touch with their bodies to become re-acquainted with sensations of tension. *The intention of contraction and relaxation was not meant in any way to fatigue the muscle. Instead, its purpose was to help recreate tension in order to become aware of subtle tension that remains after one voluntarily relaxes*. This tension, called *residual tension*, was the most important tension to release. Releasing residual tension ultimately produces the most profound relaxation.

Jacobson's main work was described in his book *Progressive Relaxation*, first published in 1929, and then revised in 1939. Throughout his lifetime he wrote books and published many articles. He was quick to point out that *Progressive Relaxation* was fundamentally different from hypnosis or psychoanalysis which were popular during his time. He had little respect for either of them. *Progressive Relaxation*, Jacobson contended, did not operate in an altered state or because of transference but in a conscious, *unaltered* state and where transference was not a factor in its effect.

One of the main points he made throughout his life was that 'the mind' was not simply found in the brain but in the peripheral muscles and nerves as well. This was the point he made in his last book, *The Human Mind*. One of the ways he demonstrated this point was by hooking subjects up to an electromyograph and asking them to imagine riding a bicycle. He found that when the subject imagined riding a bicycle, simultaneously the parts of the body involved in riding a bicycle including the hands, arms, feet and legs, subtly contracted as if the subject were actually riding. Understanding that the mind was also in the muscles of the body enabled him to control the mind by relaxing the muscles.

He introduced the then radical idea, which he demonstrated and validated objectively in his work with the relaxation of the gastrointestinal tract, that the arousal of the autonomic nervous system, long thought to be out of one's control, could be reduced voluntarily. This was a startling insight at the time.

The key to profound relaxation: the relaxation of the eyes and speech muscles

Perhaps Jacobson's greatest insight came from his discovery that visualization and conceptual thinking are always accompanied by small muscle movements of the eyes and apparatus of speech. He found that when you picture an apple in your mind, your eyes actually move and focus as if they were looking at an apple in real life. Similarly, the speech muscles, including the lips, tongue, jaw, and throat move slightly when you think in words and sentences.

The significance of this insight may escape you unless you realize that *it was Jacobson's goal to learn how to relax the muscles of the eyes and the speech apparatus as a way of stopping thought.* This quiet state of mind allows for the body to relax very deeply. The idea that you can quiet the mind by relaxing the muscles of vision and speech has been almost entirely overlooked by medicine and psychology.

As an example of the clinical usefulness of his insight, Jacobson had a patient who obsessively thought about killing her child. This obsession profoundly disturbed the woman who went to different doctors in search of help. Jacobson worked with her by helping her examine what position her eyes were in when she had this obsessive thought. He then taught her to relax her eyes and let go of inwardly looking at this image. Over time she was able to stop this obsessive thought by simply relaxing her eyes when her mind went to it. This ability to control her mind resulted in the restoration of her good mood as well as a rise in self-esteem, confidence, and long term relief from the anxiety and obsession. This *positive feedback loop* is what benefits many people who become competent in *Progressive Relaxation*. The relaxation of the eyes and speech muscles turns out to be very important in treating pelvic pain and the catastrophic thinking often associated with it.

The master skill of the adepts of meditation: quieting the eyes to stop visualization and quieting the speech muscles to stop 'inner talk'

Jacobson's discovery that relaxing the eyes and speech muscles could stop thinking is the master skill of the adepts of meditation. Over the centuries, the major wisdom traditions of the east have understood that the noisy and discursive mind blocks the experience of one's own unconditioned nature and sense of cosmic union. Certain ancient Yogic, Taoist and other esoteric meditation traditions have focused on the relaxation of the eyes and the speech muscles as a necessary preparation for accessing the deepest meditation states.

Jacobson's discovery is as simple as it is profound. One aspect of visualization is muscle activity in which the eyes focus as if they were looking at an object even though the eyes are closed. Visualization, therefore, is not only a 'mental' activity somehow separated from the body, but involves corresponding physical responses. Similarly, Jacobson found that during the process of thinking there are slight movements of the speech muscles, which he called "subvocalization." Thus thinking is a form of talking involving subtle movements of the lips, tongue, throat, and vocal cords.

When you relax the eyes and speech muscles you relax profoundly

The human organism is designed to adapt and respond to constantly changing circumstances in order to survive. All of these responses involve some degree of muscle tension. When we learn to still the mind and body and quiet the impulse to respond, we can profoundly relax and rest deeply.

We see the evidence of this in the deep rest that occurs with non-REM (non rapid eye movement) sleep (or dreamless sleep). Rapid eye movement sleep is an important aspect of a good night's rest and indicates that the person sleeping is dreaming or having visual images while sleeping. But non-REM sleep is the most restful. The most profound, restful kind of sleep occurs when there are no visual images or dreams as indicated in the absence of rapid eye movement. Absence of thought in *either* the sleeping or waking state is indicative of a state of the deepest rest.

If we have no thoughts going on in the mind, except in moments of immediate threat, there is no triggering the body's 'emergency responses' to brace and protect itself. *A profoundly quiet mind means that there is no issue about survival in that moment.*

Peace of mind means no thinking

We normally think about peace of mind as a lofty and ongoing state to be experienced on a Himalayan mountaintop or only in the experience of the old and the wise. Jacobson made the understanding of 'peace of mind' comprehensible, practical and attainable. Peace of mind means a quiet mind with no thoughts. Peace of mind allows you to relax and allows your emergency center to put the "all clear" message out. Peace of mind stops the rise of adrenalin and other stress response hormones in your blood stream allowing the body to be at peace.

The relaxation of the eyes and speech muscles is the advanced practice of Progressive Relaxation

Before you can discern the activities of your eyes and of your muscles of speech, you must learn to relax the body as a whole. Once you have established a certain level of bodily quiet, it is easier to pay attention to the stream of pictures and thoughts that cross through your mind. As you become able to witness these pictures and thoughts, you can begin the subtle practice of 'letting go of inner looking and inner talking.'

Most patients can relax the body sufficiently to reduce or stop pelvic pain and dysfunction without training in the relaxation of the eyes and speech muscles. There are some, however, who cannot become sufficiently quiet without learning this advanced skill.

Paradoxical Relaxation developed from Jacobson's work

Relaxation of muscles and quieting of the nervous system is an effect of feeling safe. This state of safety is achieved by learning to direct your attention towards accepting tension, relaxing the muscles, and stilling thoughts that trigger survival responses.

All methods of relaxation direct your attention. Some methods direct your attention to pleasing scenes. Others ask you to relax or warm your body. Jacobson asked patients to lie down and instructed them to 'discontinue effort' or 'go negative' as a way of telling them what to do with their attention in order to relax. It was his mastery of his own method that gave him such charisma and influence in the field of relaxation and autonomic self-regulation. However, his language was from the 19th century, and it is not the most useful language to communicate what we know in the twenty-first.

Jacobson tended to be brusque and patriarchal, telling his patients what to do without offering any reassurance or softness in style. In fact the very title of his book, the only one currently in print, *You Must Relax*, demonstrates the limitations of his language in communicating his insights about relaxation. Furthermore, as we have mentioned, Jacobson wanted to make sure that no one confused the success of his method with hypnosis, transference or the giving of reassurance, or because of a placebo effect. When he taught *Progressive Relaxation* to professionals, he was adamant that it was wrong for the teacher of *Progressive Relaxation* to offer any reassurance to the patient. He felt the results of relaxation should be their own reassurance. While his own view represented his high level of integrity and faith in the effectiveness of his method, instructions in relaxation associated with these considerations tend to be off-putting.

Finally, Jacobson was very concerned that his method might be regarded as some offshoot of yoga, meditation, or spiritual practice. In trying to eliminate this possible confusion, his language tended to be mechanistic, scientific, and objective—a language that often did not endear those reading his work.

During Jacobson's time, the prevailing religion was science, and any hint that a method was spiritual or mystical made the method suspect among the illuminati of the time. Jacobson shunned any hint that his method bore any relationship to so called spiritual practices. In truth, the method of *Progressive Relaxation* is in the finest tradition of the world's wisdom practices.

There was little understanding during Jacobson's time of the healing potential of acupuncture, chi gung, yoga, and meditation. This is in contrast to the present when the efficacy of these methods is well documented in the scientific literature.

We have modified the technique of *Progressive Relaxation* to make it more accessible to the modern era. We use a different language to communicate its insights and methodologies to relax the muscles of the pelvic floor. *This modification of Progressive Relaxation is what we call Paradoxical Relaxation.*

Medical monitoring in the practice of Paradoxical Relaxation

Occasionally patients may have a condition requiring medical monitoring. If you have high blood pressure, asthma, or epilepsy, you should inform the doctor who is teaching you *Paradoxical Relaxation*, as medications may need to be adjusted as you become more relaxed. For example, if someone has high blood pressure and continues the regular dose of antihypertensive medicine while more and more deeply relaxing with *Paradoxical Relaxation*, the medication may prove to be too strong for the improved state of relaxation and will need to be reduced.

What is paradoxical about Paradoxical Relaxation?

A paradox is a statement that seems to contradict itself, but nevertheless is true. Examples of paradoxes tend to be found in philosophy and spiritual writing. For example, the premise of Alcoholics Anonymous is that you can only gain control over the addiction to alcohol by admitting you are powerless over it. In the *Course of Miracles* it says, "To have, give all to all" which means that if you want something for yourself, give everything you have away. In Zen, Suzuki Roshi, a renowned Zen master wrote, "If you want a horse to be close to you, give it a big pasture."

The paradox of *Paradoxical Relaxation* is found in the relationship you train yourself to develop to your tension and is as follows; *you relax when you accept tension. The skill of individuals who are successful in profoundly relaxing the pelvic floor involves learning to be effortless in relationship to their tension and discomfort while being present with it. Paradoxical Relaxation* is the cultivation of effortlessness.

What does it mean to develop a certain relationship to your tension and discomfort? How do you become effortless in relationship to the unconscious effort that is simply another way of describing the contracted state? What does it mean to accept tension? Why would accepting tension result in relaxation? At a certain level all of this does not make sense. At another level, it speaks to the deepest truth in all of us.

As Jacobson correctly understood, relaxation has to do with letting go of effort. 'Letting go of effort' means letting go of 'doing' anything. Muscle tension generally is involved at some level in 'doing something.' This 'doing something' involves all actions we do in our life from riding a bicycle to cutting carrots. This 'doing something' may involve issues of survival, like bracing to prepare for a blow, tensing in preparation for flight, or contraction of the muscles in preparing to attack.

If we tell you to relax, your mind will probably interpret this instruction as asking that you 'do' something or make some effort, when in fact, relaxation means discontinuing effort. Relaxation means the *absence* of doing. What a peculiar idea the 'absence of doing' is. What does it mean to 'not do'?

The state of relaxation is a state of 'being.' It contains no action or volition. Notice how it feels if someone tells you to 'be.' You may find such an instruction disconcerting because generally speaking you can't do anything to 'be.'

Relaxation and 'being' are not states that you can 'make happen.' *The closest one can get to telling someone how to relax, we have discovered, is to ask them to be present with their current and immediate state without trying to change it. Our relaxation curriculum involves pointing the way to being effortless in relationship to tension. Hence we discover that when we step back and feel and accept our tension with no intention to do anything about it, after a while relaxation occurs.* Notice that we say that 'relaxation occurs' instead of saying 'you relax yourself'. Relaxation *occurs* as a natural consequence of letting go of doing. *You can't make yourself relax.*

When you accept something, you no longer exert effort in relationship to it. You let it be. When you accept your tension, you stop all conscious effort in relationship to it. This is another way of saying you relax it. This identity between acceptance and the cessation of effort in relationship to tension is the seminal insight of *Paradoxical Relaxation.*

A renowned meditation teacher, Hariwansh Lal Poonja, once said that what is *not* the state of being has been eloquently described, but *what is* the state of being has never been described. So it is with words aimed at directing someone to relax. You can say that relaxation is the stopping of doing anything, not efforting, or not trying. There are few words to say exactly what it is. *Paradoxical Relaxation* borrows from this perennial wisdom that you let go of effort by fully accepting it the way it is.

Understanding the method of Paradoxical Relaxation

The aim of Paradoxical Relaxation is to be able to allow your body to rest deeply and allow the tissue restoration and rebuilding. Its aim is to help allow your pelvis to heal from the chronic irritation of its tensed and shortened muscles and the effect of these muscles on the structures, nerves, and tissues within the pelvis. Paradoxical Relaxation is most effectively used in conjunction with the intrapelvic Myofascial/Trigger Point Release in the same way the Myofascial/Trigger Point Release is most effective when used together with Paradoxical Relaxation. Both methods need instruction by someone competent and experienced in the methods.

There are pitfalls that students of Paradoxical Relaxation can encounter of which they are often unaware. Similarly, the interior of the pelvis is not an area that someone untrained in its anatomy and physiology should enter into without the close supervision of an experienced professional. The information we share here is informational and educational, and our protocol is not intended to be a how-to method that one can use by reading this book and in the absence of competent instruction.

A fifty-five year old surgeon came to us for treatment after suffering with chronic pelvic pain syndrome for over thirty years. He was a strong and determined man who was used to doing something concrete and seeing the immediate results of his efforts.

When we first began our instruction in *Paradoxical Relaxation* he asked us how the seemingly innocuous instructions, aimed at helping him relax his pelvic muscles, could possibly make a dent in a condition that he felt had been ruining his life. His incredulity about the effects of relaxation on his condition had to be addressed so that he could practice it wholeheartedly.

In modern medical treatment we use needles, pills, creams, or scalpels against offending parts as a way of making them normal again. The idea that practicing a shift in attention onto a part of the body that is tense, and then accepting that tension, is a radical departure from the conventional medical wisdom.

Chronic tension eventually feels normal

When you learn *Paradoxical Relaxation* you focus on detecting subtle sensations of effort in your body. These sensations are unremarkable, and if someone did not tell you to pay attention to them you probably wouldn't give them any notice. Learning to relax means paying attention to the small and unremarkable efforts to which we normally pay no attention. In fact, these tensions feel normal.

A patient told us a story which illustrated the process of how tension can become what one feels to be normal. As a teenager, he went to summer camp with an odd fellow who found a pair of thick black glasses that contained no lenses. At the beginning of camp, our patient recalled, this odd fellow wore these glasses despite the disparaging and perplexed comments of other children. People told this fellow that he looked strange and asked him why he chose to wear glasses without lenses. The fellow shrugged and did not respond to the comments of others. Instead, he wore them day and night throughout the course of the summer. Eventually, people got used to him and his glasses. We can get used to almost anything.

Toward the end of the summer this fellow lost the glasses. Our patient remarked how strange it was that the very people, who disparaged these glasses at the beginning of the summer, asked this fellow what had become of his glasses toward the end of the summer. These glasses had become part of the identity of this odd fellow, and as strange as it was to others when he began wearing them, it was equally strange when he stopped.

Relearning to let go of effort

We have described how the body gets used to chronic tension in the pelvic floor. Like the glasses of this fellow, *you can get used to your chronic tension and effort*. Learning to relax requires that you be aware of your chronic states of tension. If you are not aware of this tension, it will remain with you. In acknowledging the tension you can rediscover the natural state that comes with letting go of effort in your pelvis.

When you fail to be able to relax, you usually miss the essential point that letting go of effort means accepting your unconscious refusal to let go. Letting go of effort means ceasing the attempt to change tension that doesn't easily let go. These words are often hard to understand unless you are being instructed in this on an ongoing basis by a teacher who can do it him or herself.

Relearning to come back into your body

Imagine you are given a luxurious two-hour massage in an elegant European spa. The room in which the massage takes place is soft, comfortably warm, and beautifully appointed. The masseuse is sensitive and knows what muscles allow for the easing of your tension. There are no distractions or discomforts. However, in order to fully enjoy this experience, your attention must be on the massage, not elsewhere. Your attention must be in your body or you miss the experience.

If there are areas of discomfort in the body, we tend to avoid them. This is true for pelvic pain. Your attention tends to want to focus anywhere but on the discomfort. We are programmed to pursue pleasure and avoid pain. The practice of *Paradoxical Relaxation* requires that you direct your attention back into your body even if it is initially uncomfortable to do so.

Paradoxical Relaxation and insomnia

Added to the distress of chronic pain and dysfunction, people who suffer from chronic pelvic pain commonly struggle with insomnia. Whether it is anxiety, continual pain, or nocturnal urinary frequency and urgency, many of our patients describe the havoc of being awakened several times during the night, not being able to fall back to sleep, and not getting a good night's rest.

Edmund Jacobson remarked that the quality of relaxation during the day tends to determine the quality of sleep at night. In our experience, the same is true for chronic pelvic pain. *Paradoxical Relaxation* helps with both the difficulty of falling asleep as well as with the difficulty of going back to sleep after one has awakened. Until all symptoms are *substantially* reduced, however, a good night's sleep can remain problematic.

Falling asleep tends to be easier to solve than going back to sleep. The help that *Paradoxical Relaxation* can offer in falling asleep is simple. You either follow the instructions on a relaxation tape or instructions you have memorized aimed at relaxing the body before sleep. If you have any facility in *Paradoxical Relaxation*, there is usually a high likelihood that doing this relaxation will enable you to fall asleep.

Going back to sleep

When we awake in the middle of the night, it tends to be more difficult to go back to sleep. For this reason we suggest that when you cannot go back to sleep, you get up and wake yourself fully. Sometimes splashing water on your face or walking briefly around the house helps. Upon awakening, some patients have found it useful to do the yoga-like stretches they have learned in the *Myofascial/Trigger Point Release* sessions. In addition to these exercises, specific yoga stretches sometimes can help relax the body. These stretches can take between five minutes to half an hour. Some patients go back to sleep using the current relaxation lesson they are doing. This relaxation can be done in bed. A walkman type cassette player can be used in order not to disturb one's partner.

CHAPTER 5

PARADOXICAL RELAXATION

Moment-to-Moment and Intensive Paradoxical Relaxation

In our treatment protocol we use *Paradoxical Relaxation* in two different but complementary ways. *Moment-to-Moment Paradoxical Relaxation* is used throughout your normal day to regularly interrupt the habit of tensing the pelvic muscles. Doing *Moment-to-Moment Paradoxical Relaxation* might involve 50 to100 brief relaxations during the day. As you become more skilled, this practice takes less time and is done almost automatically. The intention here is for you to abort the old, dysfunctional chronic tensing. *Intensive Paradoxical Relaxation* requires setting aside time that is devoted to the practice of the technique, without the distractions that occur during your normal everyday life. This is practiced once or twice a day with each practice period lasting a half hour to forty-five minutes.

Moment-to-Moment Paradoxical Relaxation does not offer the depth of relaxation achieved by *Intensive Paradoxical Relaxation* practice (simply referred to as *Paradoxical Relaxation*). The intensive practice represents the laboratory in which the skill of the method is developed and represents the heart of the practice. The skill of feeling, accepting, and resting with tension is honed in the *Intensive Paradoxical Relaxation* practice.

Moment-to-Moment Paradoxical Relaxation

Patients are often surprised at the number of times each day that they tense their pelvic muscles or find them in a continual state of contraction. Changing this habit is not a small matter.

Under normal circumstances most people would never be willing to devote the time and attention to change this habit. The energy required to change it comes from the strength of the desire to stop the pain and dysfunction. Most patients will devote the time and effort required to change this habit when they feel doing so reduces their symptoms. This motivation is the gift of this condition, even though it rarely feels like a gift when the symptoms exist unabated.

How to relax your pelvic muscles throughout the day

Our instruction to our patients regarding *Moment-to-Moment Paradoxical Relaxation* goes something like this, *"It is necessary that you become aware of your habit of tensing your pelvic muscles on a moment-to-moment basis and abort this habit. Throughout the day check for tension in your pelvic muscles so you can apply the technique of relaxing it. You may want to tie a string around your finger, or paste a colored piece of paper to your bathroom mirror, or paste a tiny iridescent dot on the face of your watch. Anything that you can do to remind yourself to feel your pelvic tension and relax it will help. Do this many times, as long as these mini relaxations don't interfere with your functioning during the day."*

Moment-to-moment relaxation is *not a Kegel exercise of tightening and then relaxing. Kegel exercises were originally done to strengthen weak pelvic muscles.* We generally do not believe Kegel exercises are useful with pelvic pain and, in fact, they can exacerbate symptoms.

Kegel exercises usually add tension to an already tense area in someone who has pelvic pain. Moment-to-moment relaxation involves briefly relaxing without tensing before the relaxation.

It is sometimes useful to use a small and inexpensive device called *The Motiv-Aider*. This small machine is the size of a pager and vibrates silently like someone tapping you on the shoulder at any time you designate. For instance you can set *The Motiv-Aider* (available at www.motiv-aider.com) to vibrate every ten minutes, or every hour as a private reminder to relax the pelvic muscles.

Sensing pelvic tension

It can help to become sensitive to your pelvic tension in the following the way. While you are sitting on a toilet, notice how your rectum and genitals drop and relax when you begin to urinate. These muscles naturally relax when you urinate and they tighten when you stop urination. It is these muscles that you want to learn to relax throughout the day.

Up tight and stuck up

Someone with chronic pelvic pain tends to have pelvic muscles that are held 'up' and 'tight.' The relaxed, dropped state of the pelvic muscles tends to be absent with pelvic pain. Another way to conceive of what goes on in the pelvic floor is to understand that the tight and contracted pelvic muscles are stuck in a contraction and held up in such a contraction. Hence we can describe the pelvic floor in most pelvic pain patients as 'up tight' or 'stuck up.'

It is necessary to rehabilitate this pelvic floor posture so that the default mode of the pelvic muscles is 'down' and 'relaxed.' You can practice relaxing and dropping the pelvic muscles in the following exercise. Sit on the toilet and feel the relaxation of the muscles in your pelvic floor as you begin to allow urination to occur. While still on the toilet, relax these muscles as if you are about to urinate, except do not allow yourself to urinate. Most likely, you will feel a slight dropping of the muscles around the rectum as you prepare to urinate. The muscles you relax in this exercise are the same muscles you should be relaxing with *Moment-to-Moment Paradoxical Relaxation.*

Moment-to-Moment Paradoxical Relaxation in a nutshell

Moment-to-Moment Paradoxical Relaxation is the practice of allowing the pelvic muscles to drop and relax all day. Whether you remind yourself spontaneously or are reminded by *The Motiv-Aider* or by some other means, relax and drop the pelvic muscles by noticing any pelvic tension and voluntarily relax the pelvic floor as if you are going to begin to urinate but *without* urinating. Remember that your voluntary relaxation of these muscles at first will rarely cause much of a sense of relaxation in them. It is best to expect that your voluntary relaxation will only go a little ways to relax the pelvic muscles. Nevertheless, it is important to do this relaxation on an ongoing basis until this relaxation becomes a habit that replaces the tendency of chronically tightening.

Hints on the application of the
Moment-to-Moment Paradoxical Relaxation

1. It takes time to learn

It takes time to learn how to do *Moment-to-Moment Paradoxical Relaxation* so that it does not interrupt your day. Doing it should take only a moment or two.

2. Make sure that you do not exert effort

Make sure you do not exert any effort to relax. Just as you don't exert effort to initiate urination, don't exert effort to do this momentary relaxation. Don't push down as in the Valsalva maneuver to accomplish relaxation. Instead simply imagine yourself beginning to urinate and feel the relaxation in your pelvis like you are.

3. Continue to practice even if no results seem to occur

The *Moment-to-Moment Paradoxical Relaxation* practice is aimed at subtracting tension from the pelvic muscles throughout the day.

Sometimes the effect of doing this upon symptoms is dramatic; often it is not. *We tell our patients to continue to do it whether you have results or not.*

Doing Intensive Paradoxical Relaxation

Preparation

The preparation for doing *Intensive Paradoxical Relaxation* (or simply called *Paradoxical Relaxation*) is essential for its effectiveness. Make sure that you won't be disturbed for the period of time that you are doing the relaxation. This might mean asking your spouse to make sure that your children don't come into the room in which you are relaxing. We suggest, when possible, disconnecting the telephone and turning off the television or stereo. Relaxation needs to be done with no distractions.

When possible, make sure you are choosing to do your relaxation practice at a time when you do not have an important appointment immediately afterwards that requires you to be alert and tense. Make sure your pet won't disturb you.

Bath or shower and stretches

Many people with pelvic pain are advised by their doctors to take a hot bath or a sitz bath as a way to relax the pelvic area. In fact, a warm bath or shower can be very helpful to ease pelvic discomfort. Furthermore, the warm water is a good preparation for *Paradoxical Relaxation.*

Under ideal circumstances it is helpful to take a brief warm bath or shower, do five to fifteen minutes of the stretches assigned to you by your myofascial therapist, and then do the relaxation. *While taking a bath and doing stretching prior to relaxation is advisable, it is not essential for the success of the relaxation. It simply can make the relaxation easier and deeper.*

Timer

It is best to set a timer that will ring at the end of the relaxation session. If you have fallen asleep during the relaxation period, the timer will let you know that the period is over. Because the relaxation is done first lying down, we advise the use of a pillow or two under the knees as a way of reducing stress on the lower back.

If you tend to have many things to do during the day, it is a good idea to write them down on a piece of paper so that you will have less of a tendency to carry them in your head during relaxation. Also, it is good to have a paper and pencil near you while you are doing the relaxation. If a pressing thought arises that you might have to remember, you can jot it down and continue the relaxation.

Relaxation, eating, drinking, and the bathroom

It is best not to eat any substantial amount of food prior to relaxation as it tends to make you fall asleep. While falling asleep is not bad, it is better to remain awake throughout the entire relaxation session. Furthermore, we advise patients to avoid caffeine, sugar or other stimulants.

In order to remain as comfortable as possible during the relaxation we advise people to urinate before a period of relaxation if they are feeling uncomfortable holding in the urine. Along with this, it is usually better, when possible, to avoid drinking fluids prior to relaxation, especially if you have urinary frequency and urgency. Finally, most patients are more comfortable when they loosen their tie, belt, or anything constricting.

Setting up the room

We advise patients to partially darken the room in which they are going to relax and to use an eye pillow. An eye pillow is a small sack, often made of velvet or cotton and filled with flax seed that can be bought at a health food store. It has the advantage of darkening the field of vision even in a room with a great deal of light. The eye pillow also tends to be soothing to the eyes and usually helpful for relaxation.

Paradoxical Relaxation can be done lying down or in a chair. It is advised that it be done lying down at the beginning of training, especially if there is increased pain while sitting. A bed, a couch, a futon, or a carpeted floor will work. Because the key is comfort, it is acceptable to use as many pillows as necessary.

While it is good to have a comfortable regular place for relaxation, the practice can be done almost anywhere. It is possible to do *Paradoxical Relaxation* in a hotel room, on a bus, in a plane, in your office chair, in a park on the grass, or on a towel in the sand. A personal portable headphone-stereo, such as a Walkman, makes listening to the instructions on the relaxation tapes private and accessible, even in the most public of places.

What about falling asleep?

It is not uncommon to fall asleep during *Paradoxical Relaxation*. Falling asleep is more likely if you are tired and if you do the relaxation during a part of the day when you tend to become fatigued, as in the afternoon or evening.

Falling asleep is of little concern, especially in the beginning of relaxation training. It is preferable to allow yourself to doze rather than to tense for the purpose of staying awake. The experience of sleep during *Paradoxical Relaxation* tends to be different from simply falling asleep at other times. If you fall asleep almost all of the time, try sitting up and making sure that the room you are in is not overly warm. If you are in treatment and do relaxation to go to sleep, we suggest that this *not* be counted as a period of practice. An additional session would need to be done to comply with our protocol.

The best time to do Paradoxical Relaxation

The best time to do Paradoxical Relaxation is when you have the most energy. Most people find that they have this kind of energy in the morning. However, this is not universally true. Some people have more energy and ability to pay attention in the afternoon.

The reason energy is required for *Paradoxical Relaxation* is that you are attempting to modify a habit of inner tension that has been practiced countless times. Establishing a new habit in the face of such a practiced habit is ambitious. It is for this reason that each practice period must 'really count' by virtue of the earnestness and level of attention with which it is done.

It is best to get into a routine doing *Paradoxical Relaxation* so the body gets used to a regular time of quiet. A routine also helps avoid missing relaxation sessions. While we normally advise people to do *Paradoxical Relaxation* at least once a day, when possible it is good to do it twice a day. The best times tend to be in the morning and afternoon or evening, but before a major meal.

Summary

- Go to the bathroom prior to relaxation to be as comfortable as possible in your pelvis
- If possible, take a warm bath and/or do the stretches immediately prior to beginning relaxation
- Make sure you are comfortable and will not be disturbed
- If possible, darken room or use eye pillow
- Set a timer
- Have a pen and paper by your side
- Avoid caffeine, stimulants, and sedatives
- Do relaxation when you have the most energy
- It is better to do relaxation in imperfect conditions than not at all

Beginning Paradoxical Relaxation

After the Respiratory Sinus Arrhythmia (RSA) breathing, which we will soon discuss, the cassette recordings of *Paradoxical Relaxation* instruction have made the practice relatively simple. All of the instructions for the practice are provided in the thirty-six lessons in the taped series. A small cassette player with a headset that goes over the ears is usually used. Noise-canceling headphones, like ones' from PlaneQuiet or Bose are useful when the relaxation method can be used on a plane or in a noisy place.

Follow the instructions on the tapes earnestly

The primary purpose of using the cassette training tapes is to repetitively hear the instructions about the subtle practice of accepting tension so that the instructions become automatic. There is a natural tendency for your attention to wander when you repeatedly hear something. The practice of accepting tension is not generally something you learn quickly. The habits of letting your attention wandering and the old tensions returning will continue to reassert themselves.

Listen to the instructions on the tapes carefully each time you do the relaxation. Follow them as closely as you can. If you don't understand an instruction, ask your instructor to clarify it. When you feel and accept tension the body tends to relax. Below we discuss the subtle aspects of *Paradoxical Relaxation.*

Daily checklist

Patients are asked to keep a record of their experience during the relaxation. Over a period of time the answers to the checklist provide an understanding of the effect of the relaxation upon symptoms.

Daily Checklist for Paradoxical Relaxation Training

Do item 1 before the relaxation session and the rest of the questions after your session

Name_____ Date_____ Session #_____

Number of tape you are listening to _____

1. Global symptom level before relaxation
   0   1   2   3   4   5   6   7   8   9   10
   (No discomfort)   (Worst discomfort)

2. Global symptom level after relaxation
   0   1   2   3   4   5   6   7   8   9   10
   (No discomfort)   (Worst discomfort)

3. At what time did you do the relaxation?

4. Did you fall asleep during relaxation?
       Yes   No

   If yes, approximately what percentage of the relaxation period were you asleep? _____%

5. Were you alone and undisturbed by outside factors?
       Yes   No

   If no, describe disturbance _____

6. Did you understand the instructions on the tape?
       Yes   No

   If no, explain _____

7. What did you do well during relaxation? With what did you have difficulty?

8. Is the concept of accepting tension /resting with tension clear to you?

      Yes   No

      If no, explain _____

9. What level of success have you had in accepting or resting with tension?

10. Did you listen to the entire tape?

      Yes   No

11. How intrusive was the pain/discomfort in your pelvis when you were doing the relaxation?

      Very intrusive_____   Somewhat intrusive_____
      Slightly intrusive_____   Not intrusive_____

12. How closely are you listening to the instructions on during the relaxation?

      Very closely____   Somewhat closely_____   Not closely____

13. Questions/comments

Accepting tension to relax can seem counter-intuitive

All of the instructions of Paradoxical Relaxation provide ways in which we assist you to remember how to let go of effort. True relaxation is a state of effortlessness. Most of us can remember times in our lives when we felt peaceful and happy. In those times there tended to be no trace of strain, tension, or effort. Those times felt easy. The experience most patients have is not one of effortlessness or ease, and yet it is what patients most deeply yearn for.

Relaxation = feeling and accepting tension

You will discover how relaxation results from feeling and accepting tension by giving yourself this instruction and seeing how it impacts you. We have found that using the instructions 'feel and accept tension' or 'feel the tension without trying to do anything about it' are a few of the phrases in our repertoire of instruction in teaching someone to cease efforting. It is important to note that the method of *Paradoxical Relaxation* asks the patient to make a distinction between pain and tension. While pain needs to be acknowledged and not resisted, the focus of our methodology is on focusing on tension as foreground and not pain as foreground. An experienced teacher can help the student of *Paradoxical Relaxation* understand this essential distinction.

How can the accepting of tension offer the possibility of deep relaxation?

The Example of Riding a Bicycle

Accepting tension is like learning to ride a bicycle. Let's imagine you have never ridden a bicycle and we present you with a simple balloon-tire, old-style, or a one-speed bicycle. We can say, "Put your leg over the bicycle and sit on the seat and push off with one leg while the other leg is in the stirrup of the other pedal and when you start falling to the left, lean to the right, and when you start falling to the right, lean to the left."

For those of us who can ride a bicycle, it is clear that these instructions will not go very far in teaching you how to ride a bicycle. The best way to learn how to ride a bicycle is to get on one and ride it. Knowing this, parents will often teach their children how to ride a bicycle by letting them get on the bicycle while the parent runs long side of it and holds it upright. Training wheels are sometimes used as a replacement for the parent running alongside the child.

The example of riding a bicycle makes it obvious that the only way you learn is ultimately by doing. Instructions may be helpful, but do not substitute for actually being in the seat of the bicycle and having to contend with the forces that are pulling you off balance at every moment. While it is helpful to have a coach who is practiced in the skill you wish to master, all such skills are ultimately learned through direct experience. So it is with *Paradoxical Relaxation*.

The experience of accepting tension

Get comfortable

While reading this section, make sure that you are comfortable. If it is uncomfortable for you to sit, it is fine to recline as you do this exercise. It is sometimes useful to begin the practice of *Paradoxical Relaxation* by quieting the nervous system using what we call RSA breathing described below.

Respiratory Sinus Arrhythmia breathing (RSA breathing) in preparation for Paradoxical Relaxation

RSA breathing is a description of the relationship between heart rate and breathing and refers to the heart rate varying in response to respiration. RSA is a phenomenon that occurs in all vertebrates. You can experience the phenomenon of RSA by taking your pulse and noting that when you breathe in, the heart rate increases slightly and when you breathe out the heart rate decreases slightly. There is considerable research that indicates that when there is balance and health, the heart rate and the breath move robustly together as inhalation occurs, heart rate increases as exhalation occurs, heart rate drops.

Under circumstances of mental or physical disease the relationship between breathing and heart rate is disturbed. When individuals suffer panic attacks for instance, RSA is lower and is disturbed. When they recover from panic disorders their RSA breathing becomes stronger, more balanced, and robust. The higher and stronger the heart rate variability is in relationship to appropriate respiration, the higher is the general at a level of health and well being. For example healthy children generally have very robust RSA breathing in which the heart rate can sometimes vary 40 beats or more between inhalation and inhalation.

Reduced RSA is thought to be an indicator of an adverse prognosis for people with heart disease. Generally disturbed RSA is indicative of early problems in the healthy functioning of the autonomic nervous system as it relates to a number of diseases. It has been suggested that one measure of the therapeutic effect or safety of a drug is whether it positively or negatively affects RSA.

It is usually possible with certain breathing protocols to voluntarily change the RSA and bring it into balance. Restoring RSA can facilitate autonomic quieting and a reduction of anxiety in consciously coordinating the heart rate and respiration. We use this practice as part of *Paradoxical Relaxation.*

RSA focused breathing should be done under the supervision of a professional. Occasionally, RSA can trigger benign ectopic or missed heart beats. Lightheadedness or a sense of not getting enough air can occur when the correct technique is not used. If there are any problems that occur such as lightheadedness or not getting enough air during the RSA breathing, you should consult with the doctor who is teaching you the method about adjusting your breathing and correcting your technique. Otherwise, RSA can be a useful method to quickly quiet sympathetic nervous system arousal, reduce anxiety, and allow one to be at a deeper level of relaxation when beginning the practice of accepting tension which is the heart of the relaxation method discussed here.

Practicing RSA breathing

It is generally agreed that slow abdominal breathing in which the abdomen rises during inhalation and falls back during exhalation is important in relaxation of the body and in the reduction of autonomic arousal. Slow abdominal breathing maximizes the possibility of breathing and heart rate coming into synchrony with each other. While there is no formula rigidly defining how many respirations per minute should occur for deep relaxation to occur, 6 deep abdominal breaths per minute is more or less considered an optimal respiration rate. Again 6 breaths per minute is an ideal and breathing rates that accomplish preliminary quieting of the body can vary from 2 to 9 breaths per minute depending on idiosyncrasies and experience of the particular patient. More important than having an idea of what the ideal number of breaths per minute should be is the understanding that one's level of comfort in breathing is the most important criteria in fine tuning one's respiration rate. If you are slowing your breath to approximately 6 breaths per minute, as we will describe below, you should adjust this slower respiration rate up or down to fit your individual level of comfort.

Computing the number of heart beats per breath in RSA breathing

In *Paradoxical Relaxation*, RSA breathing is sometimes done for 10 to 20 minutes immediately prior to following the instruction on the taped audio course. Below are the instructions about doing RSA breathing. To determine how many heartbeats you will devote to inhalation and how many heartbeats you will devote to exhalation, use the following computations (these computations may appear to make the technique more complicated than it is). After proper instruction from someone experienced in RSA breathing, the following instructions can serve as a guide.

1. Take your pulse and determine how many times your heart beats per minute. Feeling the pulse in the wrist with three fingers gently pressed on the side of the wrist closest to the thumb is one of the easiest ways to determine your heart rate. Counting how many heart beats occur in a 15 second time frame and then multiplying that number by 4 is an easy way to determine your pulse rate per minute.

2. Divide your heart rate by 6. If for instance you have a heart rate of 60 beats per minute the computation would be:

$$\frac{60}{6} = 10$$ (Represents the number of beats allocated for a full in and out breath in order to breath 6 times per minute)

Divide 10 by 2 = 5 (Represents the number heartbeats allocated for a single inhalation or exhalation)

Likewise, if you have a heart rate of 72 beats per minute, 72 divided by 6 = 12, and 12 divided by 2 = 6.

3. Lie down preparing to do *Paradoxical Relaxation* with your lesson on tape queued up on the tape player and ready to play. Be in a position so that you are physically comfortable for 10 minutes in following your heart rate by resting your hands over your heart or comfortably feeling your pulse in your wrist. Sometimes pillows can be placed under the elbows of both arms to feel the pulse in the wrist and to reduce the tension in the arms and hands while feeling the heart rate. This makes it easier to feel the pulse on an ongoing basis for 15 minutes.

4. Once you are relaxed and feeling your pulse comfortably, count up to 5 heart beats (if your heart rate is 60, as in the example above) as you inhale raising your abdomen and then count to 5 heartbeats as you exhale. If your heart rate is 72, you would could up to 6 beats as you inhale or exhale.

5. You can vary the amount of air you breathe. If you are feeling that you are not getting enough air, breathe more air. If you feel uncomfortable getting too much air, reduce your air intake.

6. You can breathe in or out more quickly at the beginning, middle or end of the count of 5, depending on what feels comfortable.

7. It is most important that your breathing is *comfortable*. Your comfort level is the most important fact in considering to breathe more or less air or more quickly or slowly at any given part of the breathing cycle. As in *Paradoxical Relaxation*, bring your attention back over and over again to the sensation of the breath, away from attending to visual or conceptual thinking.

8. Continue to breathe in and out to the count of your allocated number of heartbeats bringing your attention away from thinking to the sensation of the breath. When your breathing feels uncomfortable, adjust it by taking in less air or more air or by breathing more quickly or slowly at the beginning, middle or end of the either the inhalation or exhalation. Your job is to make sure your breathing is comfortable in breathing 6 times per minute. If it is easier to breathe 7 beats or 4 beats per inhalation or exhalation, make the adjustment (more beats per breath slows down the breathing rate, fewer beats increase the breathing rate). Comfort is the first priority.

9. Continue the RSA breathing for 10 minutes. Mark the end of the RSA breathing by setting an alarm for this time. Then begin the *Paradoxical Relaxation* without regulating your breath at all.

RSA breathing and quieting down urinary frequency and urgency

Some patients have reported that the practice of the RSA breathing has quieted down the urge to urinate. We have no systematic study of this but for instance a patient who felt the urge to urinate a few minutes after he had urinated and was stuck on an airplane runway and had to remain seated for an hour did the RSA breathing and reported that he was able to almost stop his sense of urinary urgency. Others have reported that they have been able to use skin rolling (discussed later) to accomplish this. Both the RSA breathing and the skin rolling are easy and safe to do and may be able to help patients mange their symptoms a little more easily.

Relax the sides of your face

After RSA breathing for approximately 10 minutes, relax your hands that have been monitoring your pulse and let go of controlling your breath. Let your breathing be entirely unregulated as you breathe comfortably.

Having let go of controlling your breathing, close your eyes, and feel your face muscles. Relax the sides of your face. Let go of the muscles that you use to 'put a face on' in the world. When your attention wanders, as it inevitably will, bring it back to feeling the sensations in the sides of your face.

Find a part of your body that is tense (not in the pelvis)

Now find a part of the body that feels tense. It does not have to be any great or unbearable tension, just a simple sensation of tension. Tension in the shoulders or neck, however unremarkable, is a suitable area to focus on for the purpose of this exercise.

It is less helpful in this exercise to focus on tension in the pelvic floor since it is often highly emotionally charged, with great attachment to the area feeling better. This strong attachment, especially to the beginner, makes the practice of accepting tension more difficult.

Inwardly locate the tension

The outside world is familiar to us when we open our eyes and look across the room or across the street. If we are asked where the street corner is, we will easily locate it and point it out. If we were to ask you to look at your left knee, you would not have any trouble in finding it. If we were to ask you to locate your right hand, you would not have any difficulty in locating it.

The inner world of sensation, thought, and emotion is not so clear. When you close your eyes and notice a sensation of tension, while its location may be clear in your mind, it usually does not have the discreet boundaries and precise location that occur when you see your hand with your eyes open. In learning *Paradoxical Relaxation*, we need practice in locating sensation inside the body. Tensing and relaxing a part of the body is designed to teach us to locate the body tensions while the eyes are closed.

Bring your attention again inside your body and again find a part of the body that is tense. Direct your attention to this tension. Tense and then relax this part of the body. Feel it. Now allow it to exist as you originally felt it without trying to change it or do anything to it.

There is a quality of attention that can help you more clearly locate and relax the tension in your body. While feeling this tension now, be more receptive than active in perceiving it. *Let the sensation come toward you rather than you reaching out toward it.*

To best achieve this receptive attitude it is important to be steady with your attention. To practice doing this now, feel the tension in your body without trying to define its borders or its exact location inside you. It is as if you have a camera you are looking through. You point the camera in the approximate direction of the object you want to photograph. Let us imagine that this camera automatically focuses once the camera is pointed in a certain direction and held still there. After a few moments, while the camera rests in a state of semi focus, its automatic focuser brings the object into focus.

Your attention works like this camera. Point your attention at your tension and practice sustaining it there. Give your attention a chance to focus in on the tension. Be patient. Don't be concerned about gaining a sense of the precise boundaries of the tension. Let the sensation of the tension come to you like the smell of jasmine comes to you on a warm summer night. You don't have to grab the scent of the jasmine. It finds its way to you; so does the sensation of tension.

Let your attention rest on this tense area

To accept tension, start out by simply feeling the sensations of the tension. These sensations are usually unremarkable. If someone didn't tell you to notice the sensation of tension in your neck or shoulders for instance, it is very unlikely you ever would bother. Again, bring your attention to the tension you have chosen, and feel it. You don't have to do anything about the tension. Just feel it. Do that now.

Direct your attention to sensation and not thought or mental pictures

It is essential to become practiced in *directly feeling* the sensation of tension and not focusing on visualizing a picture or thinking a thought of it. When you slip into a warm fragrant bath, you probably will directly feel the warmth and support of the bath and smell the fragrance in it. The bath experience is a sensory one and not an intellectual one.

The practice of *Paradoxical Relaxation* requires that you focus on *sensation* directly. When your attention wanders to thoughts in the form of sentences and pictures in your mind, gently bring your attention back to the experience of the sensation. *Getting good at Paradoxical Relaxation means getting good at keeping your attention on sensation and quickly returning to sensation when your mind wanders into thinking.* Disciplining the attention to remain one pointed in accepting the experience of the sensation of tension is 90% of the skill of this method. There is no royal road—practice, practice and more practice is the secret.

Continue to spend a few minutes focusing on a part of your body you have chosen. Feel and accept the tension. In accepting the tension you feel, you may be able to get a sense of the task involved in learning *Paradoxical Relaxation.*

Common Difficulties
People Have in Accepting Tension

How can you tell the difference between paying attention to sensation as opposed to thinking?

When you correctly bring your attention to sensation, your mind will become quiet and there will tend to be a reduction of images or sentences going through your mind. When you pay attention to sensation, you have to be in the present, neither going back to the past, nor considering the future. Thoughts may flit in and out, but your attention will be on the sensations you are feeling. When your attention shifts to thinking, you will usually feel a slight increase in tension and discomfort.

During *Paradoxical Relaxation*, attending to the sensations of tension is often interspersed with awareness of fleeting thoughts. Stay connected to *feeling* sensation, and continue to bring your attention away from the thoughts.

The following metaphor can be useful in understanding how to keep attention focused on sensation rather than on thoughts. See yourself walking down a crowded city sidewalk. Many people are walking in the opposite direction. Many faces (ideas) come toward you and pass behind as they continue in the opposite direction. If you are clear about where you are going, you continue in your direction (feeling the sensation). While you may see many of the faces through the periphery of your vision, you don't stop to have conversations with these people. You simply go in your direction.

Do the same thing with the thoughts that cross your awareness as you focus on feeling the sensations of tension. It is fine to be aware of them as they pass, but stay connected to your focus on feeling sensation without stopping and getting involved or carried away with these thoughts.

Accepting tension includes feeling and accepting your resistance to accepting tension

As you continue to rest your attention on the sensation of tension, you may notice an aversion or resistance to doing this. If this resistance or aversion could talk it might say, "Hey, this is no fun. This does not feel good. I don't like it. I want to move. I want to feel better. I want to do something. Yuck! I want to get out of here!"

This resistance is normal. The human organism is not programmed to focus on discomfort or tension. It is programmed to move toward pleasure and away from pain.

Unless you include this resistance in your sphere of acceptance, it will stalemate you. The unacknowledged resistance stays put as long as it is unacknowledged and unaccepted. In acknowledging and accepting the resistance, you open the door for it to leave.

What to do with pain or discomfort while doing Paradoxical Relaxation

We mentioned earlier that it is important for the practitioner of *Paradoxical Relaxation* to be able to make the distinction between pain/discomfort and tension. If, for instance, you are focusing on and accepting the tension in your neck and shoulders, you may have your pelvic pain or tension intrude in your focus on your neck and shoulders. If you imagine that you are speaking to someone, and in the background there is a person wearing a very loud colored shirt that is drawing your attention, continue to speak to the person, but *allow the fact that the loud colored shirt* of the person in the background *is intruding itself in your awareness and distracting you.* The practice we are suggesting is this. Don't try to block the colored shirt out of your awareness. Instead, continue your conversation (i.e., your focus on your tension) and include the colored shirt (i.e., the pain or discomfort) and also include and allow your own disturbance and distraction by it.

In summary, if there is pain or discomfort in your pelvis or elsewhere, we teach you to allow these sensations but let them be in the background of your awareness. If pain intrudes in your awareness, allow it but continue to focus on the tension. Let the pain be in the background while letting the tension upon which you are focusing be foreground. Exert no effort in relationship to your own contraction against these sensations. Accept these sensations as you accept the tension. Accept them all as sensation and not as a concept or as a visual image.

Making the distinction between pain/discomfort and tension and focusing on the tension

As one's ability to focus improves, relaxing the pelvic floor directly becomes possible (it is not a good idea to try to relax the painful or tense pelvic floor muscles in the beginning of the relaxation training). It is important when relaxing the pelvic floor or any other part of the body in which one feels discomfort, to distinguish between the sensation of tension and the sensation of pain or discomfort. The tension usually feels tight, closed, gripping, squeezed or contracted. The pain or discomfort can feel burning, torn, raw, ripped, hot or achy. When doing *Paradoxical Relaxation* while focusing on a painful area, focus on the tension while allowing the painful sensations to exist in your awareness without blocking them out or defending against them.

In relaxing a tense and painful pelvic floor, it is as if you are having a conversation with one person while the person's partner right beside you is jumping up and down. Acknowledge and allow the jumping up and down of the person while continuing your dialogue with the person to whom you are talking. Feel and accept the sensation of tension while allowing, but not focusing on, attending to, or trying to influence, the sensation of pain or discomfort. If the pain or discomfort reduces while you are relaxing, that is fine. If it does not relax, that is also fine.

It is as if you are saying to your tension and pain, "I feel you, tension, and I feel you, pain. I am focusing my attention on the tension now. You are not remarkable, tension. However, I am feeling you now. I feel you, pain, as well. I wish you weren't here. I want you to stop. However, I am going to include you in my experience and allow you to be here along with my desire to get rid of you. I am doing my best not to tense up against you or push you away. I am allowing you to be here now, but I am paying attention to feeling and accepting the tension."

Nowhere to go, nothing to do, no goal to achieve

As you feel the tension now, remember that there is nothing to achieve. *Our instructions here are simple; feel the sensations of tension and all the resistances that arise in doing this without fixing on a goal of relaxation.* Notice that when you find yourself just *hanging out* with your tension, your conditioning and natural inclination may be to 'do something' about it.

It is important to remain aware of the inclination to do something about the tension you are feeling. In the beginning of *Paradoxical Relaxation* people sometimes report feeling restless which may incline them to want to wiggle or move to relieve their sense of uneasiness in the tension. In the first few minutes of relaxation, we usually suggest that the patient allow this wiggling or movement. After these few minutes, do your best to notice the impulse to move, and notice the tension related to this impulse, but focus on the tension you feel. Following this inclination to move, to want to 'do something,' may interfere with learning to relax the tensions by accepting them. Your job is to feel these tensions associated with wanting to move, just like you have been doing with the other tensions.

Continue to feel the tension on which you have chosen to focus

You may notice that the tension subsides as you continue to feel and accept it. You may feel this as a kind of easing. If tension in your shoulders is your focus, you may notice the shoulders drop slightly.

This experience of relaxation (or the easing of the tension) tends to regularly occur when you accept tension. You may find that as this tension eases, a new and lower level of tension appears. It is like opening one door and walking down a hallway to discover another closed door. This second closed door is the natural reaction of the body to resist sudden precipitous change.

Understood in this way, the new lower level of tension is simply a way station along the way to complete relaxation. It is the body saying "Okay, I can let go, but I can't let go all the way right now—so I'll let down a little."

The tension you are accepting is dynamic and changes and shifts regularly

When you hold a baby, you will often be aware of the baby's squirming and movement in your arms. The experienced and loving parent knows to hold the baby loosely but firmly, allowing the squirming when it occurs, but keeping a solid hold on the baby.

Accepting tension is like holding a baby. The tension will usually move and shift over and over again. Doing *Paradoxical Relaxation* involves holding or allowing the shifting and squirming of the tension as you attend to it and accept it. Remember the tension is your unconscious holding. You are focusing on and accepting your own holding. This holding at first doesn't know what to do with such attention, as it is used to your resistance to it. Allow your tension or unconscious holding to simply be there, and allow it to move and shift, release and tighten, relax and squirm. Be present with you tension and accept it like you would be present with, hold and accept the squirming of your beloved infant.

Grasping for more

What often happens when one door opens only to find another is that the desire for complete relief is ignited. We could call this desire a grasping for pleasure and relief which results in increased tension. You move from an inner attitude of openness and allowing to an attitude that is not in harmony with the fact of the inner closed door. Any grasping necessarily involves increased tension.

When you are able to feel the relaxation of tension without becoming attached to more, you can relax very deeply, very quickly. There is no secret to doing this. Follow the instruction of accepting whatever tension arises at whatever level. This is a practice of postponing gratification. And paradoxically, the result is an increase in gratification in the form of deeper and deeper relaxation.

You give it up to get it

Our purpose for doing *Paradoxical Relaxation* is to achieve profound relaxation of the pelvic muscles. *Understanding this principle and orienting your attention toward relaxation of your muscles will allow you a level of relaxation not available otherwise.*

Pay attention to the moments when you are trying to manipulate yourself to relax by accepting tension

The key to accepting tension involves *sincerely* accepting tension. Notice when you have not sincerely committed yourself to accepting your tension. Most of us don't want to give up our grasping. Most people go through a stage of trying to manipulate themselves to be in a state of acceptance of tension, while not truly inhabiting that intention. You can't pretend to accept tension and experience the fruits of a sincere acceptance of tension.

When there is a part of you that refuses to sincerely accept the tension, that refusal can be felt as additional tension and discomfort. This refusal exists in most of us, and is a problem only if it is unrecognized and the tension of it unaccepted. In other words, feel the tension that is part of the refusal to sincerely accept your tension. What we are talking about here may make little sense to you without doing *Paradoxical Relaxation*.

The effort error

Dr. Edmund Jacobson described failure to understand the principle of 'giving it up to get it' as the 'effort error.' Jacobson described relaxation as the practice of 'letting go of effort.' *Any attempt 'to relax,' which is understood to mean doing anything, is trying to use effort to discontinue effort. Efforting to stop effort does not work.*

Accepting tension is letting go of effort

When you simply feel and accept tension you are practicing the essence of relaxation. When we instruct you to feel the tension we mean to let the tension be there without adding to or subtracting anything from it. When we say *rest with the tension* we are instructing you to feel the tension and do your best to quiet yourself down while experiencing it. You are not trying to change the tension and there is no effort involved. This effortlessness allows for relaxation.

Imagine that you are lying directly on a wood floor without any pillows or blankets and you have not had any sleep in two days. You are completely exhausted and can hardly keep your eyes open. Now imagine that you are right on the edge of falling asleep. At that moment your muscles relax even though you are aware of the hardness of the wood.

You can consider your tension in the same way as you consider the wood floor. You are intimately connected with the tension as you are intimately in contact with the wood floor. In accepting tension you are allowing yourself to rest deeply on the wood floor of your tension. *The difference between resting on the wood floor and resting with tension is that in resting with the tension, the tension itself will tend to relax as well.*

Accepting 'what is'

When you accept tension or discomfort you are neither adding anything to nor subtracting anything from the discomfort. You are 'laying alongside' the tension. You are not doing anything to it except being present and feeling it.

The Japanese form of poetry known as Haiku demonstrates the pure intention to accept 'what is.' Here are some examples:

> *Crisp autumn leaves*
> *Rustle softly*
> *Then blow away*

> *A red hawk glides*
> *With no effort and no sound*
> *Near a white cloud*

> *Warm fragrant air*
> *Fills the valley floor*
> *In the lush tree a blue bird squawks*

In these poems the poet simply reports his experience of what is in front of him. There is no embellishment, no judgment, and no interpretation to what is perceived. The poet reports what is directly.

Be patient with yourself. It takes practice to be present with discomfort. The more you are able to accept the discomfort without judging it, interpreting it, or trying to change it in any way, the better. *Whatever arises in your awareness as you feel your tension and discomfort, continue to apply the basic instruction of feeling and then accepting what arises. This allows for the deepest relaxation.*

Applying the basic instruction to whatever arises

In the practice of *Paradoxical Relaxation* we offer you a strategy for dealing with the fear and aversion that can arise when you are relaxing with your discomfort. Instead of being focused on and distracted by the fear or aversion, we suggest you simply allow these feelings to be present in your experience. Coexist with them. Hang out with them. Allow whatever arises.

Staying focused

The wisdom traditions of the East often discuss the necessity of strengthening the mind as a requisite for experiencing the most subtle aspects of reality. This 'strength of mind' refers to the ability to concentrate without the wavering of attention.

When you first begin *Paradoxical Relaxation* you will probably have some difficulty in staying focused. While this can be disconcerting, it is normal. There is no royal road to staying focused. The ability to stay focused, like any ability, comes with practice. *When your mind wanders from its focus, return it to the sensation of tension again and again.* It can take a month or two of regular practice to gain some competence in beginning to manage this wavering of your mind. Persevere. Don't be discouraged by the number of times you find your mind wandering.

Your tension responds to your unconditional acceptance in the same way that you respond to someone else's unconditional acceptance

Imagine you spend time with somebody who accepts you unconditionally. Imagine they communicate to you their commitment in the following way:

"I want to be present with you exactly as you are. I am not asking you to change in any way. While I may have preferences about how I might want you to be, I am committed to letting go of those preferences in favor of letting you be exactly the way you are. You may change from one moment to the next, and I am committed to being fully present with you on a moment-to-moment basis and to feel and accept you however much you change. No matter what happens in this moment, I am determined to let you be as you are with an open and sincere heart."

Most people would be very grateful to have a friend like this. When someone is present with us like this, we can relax. There is no danger of attack or judgment. The organism's emergency systems can rest, for there is no need to defend or to ensure survival. No need for vigilance. The attitude of such a friend is true support.

The tissues of your body respond to this unconditional attitude as you do. Your tissues are imbued with your intelligence. The tissue has the same consciousness as you do. It recognizes the presence of such an accepting attitude.

Most people are looking for relationships in which they are regarded in this unconditional way. In *Paradoxical Relaxation* you are asked to be this kind of friend to yourself.

Presence

Paradoxical Relaxation cannot be effectively done without your full presence. This means that as you feel the tension you remain present with it. When you find yourself distracted by thoughts of the past or future, return your attention to this present moment. *Practice returning from daydreaming over and over again.*

Now, now, now and more now

Be present now. Feel the tension now. Rest with the tension now. Take your mind back from wandering now. Feel the tension without interfering with it now. Accept the tension now. All of the instructions in *Paradoxical Relaxation* are intimately tied to now. *Paradoxical Relaxation* only works as your attention is here and now. Relaxation of your pelvic muscles occurs in the *now*.

As we have said, the commitment to keeping your attention in the present moment often flies against the ingrained habits of thought that carry you back and forth from the past to the future. Being in this present moment often requires that you experience the discomfort and dysfunction that is the hallmark of pelvic pain. *It is the commitment to keeping your attention in the present moment that can allow the undoing of the discomfort and dysfunction.* While doing relaxation, forget the past and be present now. Forget the future and be present now. Hear every instruction in *Paradoxical Relaxation* as including the word *now*.

Faith and patience

Practicing *Paradoxical Relaxation* is practicing patience. The famous trio—Crosby, Stills and Nash, sang a famous lyric, "If you can't be with the one you love, love the one you are with." In *Paradoxical Relaxation* 'the one we love' is ease and comfort. 'The one we are with' is tension and discomfort. Being present with 'the one we are with' and letting go of grasping for 'the one we love' cannot be done without patience. We tell our patients that our treatment is the 'slow fix' not the 'quick fix.' This slow fix requires the postponement of gratification.

There are inevitably many ups and downs. Flare-ups are simply part of the process. We advise our patients not to celebrate when they feel better, nor to despair when they feel worse.

Paradoxical Relaxation is not taking a nap: it is a great royal battle

When you take a nap, you let go of controlling your attention… you relax and let your attention go wherever it likes. And you fall asleep. In *Paradoxical Relaxation* you are actively controlling your attention. The point is not to fall asleep. The attention of the novice at *Paradoxical Relaxation* is usually undisciplined. Focusing this attention is not easy and the beginner quickly notices how easily his or her attention is distracted. Often hundreds of time during relaxation, the beginner has to redirect attention away from thinking and daydreaming, back to the effortless attention on the sensation of the remaining tension.

Paradoxical Relaxation, in large part, is attention training. It is the practice of controlling attention. Ramana Maharshi, one of the great sages, described meditation as a *royal battle* in which one fights to keep one's attention on the object of meditation. As one gets used to keeping attention focused, there is less struggle and eventually, as one gets to taste the fruits of controlled attention, the battle ends and the attention willingly and easily rests in sensation.

Why We Don't Sell Stand-alone Relaxation Tapes

At the time of the third printing of our book, we use a 36-lesson, year and a half course on cassette tape as part of our home course in *Paradoxical Relaxation*. While many people have contacted us about buying these tapes, it has been our experience over the years that using the relaxation course on a stand-alone basis is not effective without personal instruction by someone competent in the method. Below is a response, published on the internet, to the question of selling the relaxation tapes on a stand-alone basis.

(Part of David Wise's reply, revised for the third edition of *A Headache in the Pelvis*, to the webmaster of the ChronicProstatitis.org chat group responding to the question of selling the recorded Paradoxical Relaxation course on a stand alone basis.)

> "....I do not sell the audio *Paradoxical Relaxation* course on a stand-alone basis. There are numerous relaxation tapes that can be bought from many different sources and people are free to buy them. I could sell the recorded relaxation course I use on a stand-alone basis. I have certainly had enough requests, but choosing not to do this is neither a casual nor a self-serving decision on my part. I have a short answer and a long answer to explain why."

> *Here is the short answer.* I have no confidence that someone can learn to relax a painful pelvic floor from a relaxation tape without

both instruction from someone who is competent in the method himself or herself and without pelvic *Myofascial/Trigger Point Release*. There are patients who have gotten a hold of earlier tapes in the recorded relaxation training course and have attempted to learn the protocol by listening to the tapes without competent instruction. Sometimes a physical therapist who has copies of these earlier lessons gives a copy of these tapes to a patient and says "here are some tapes to try." The patient goes home and listens to these tapes for a while, comes up against some difficulty and usually abandons their use. The tapes wind up on the shelf and the patient is convinced that relaxation of the pelvic floor isn't possible. This is a great shame in my opinion. It closes off what I believe is a critical component in recovering from pelvic pain. I speak from my own experience and many patients that I have treated.

Like learning the piano or learning carpentry you need a real teacher who is a true pianist or carpenter. Taped recordings of relaxation instruction without the communication of the skilled teacher to the earnest student usually fails. Furthermore, you can only teach someone to go as far as you yourself can go with any skill particularly with the profound relaxation of the pelvic floor. I don't support anyone teaching *Paradoxical Relaxation* who is not skilled in it and who does not do it regularly him or herself.

I had the best teachers in relaxation, including having the privilege of working with Edmund Jacobson for a number of years, and even with such support and access to unequalled instruction, learning relaxation was hugely difficult and took me years to learn. There is no quick way here. I know this personally. I do not want to associate myself with making available a half measure that appears to offer something substantial but does not.

When I was symptomatic, I tried many remedies that all seemed reasonable but ultimately failed to help me. They left me hopeful at first, then disappointed, and disheartened. A stand-alone relaxation tape, in my opinion, is a half measure. Half measures give little chance of offering real recovery from chronic pelvic pain syndromes. I have decided that if I am to err, I will err in the direction of not offering anything instead of offering a half measure in which I have no confidence.

Here is the long answer. Learning to deeply relax the pelvic muscles in order to facilitate the healing of a sore and contracted pelvic floor from a relaxation tape that you buy, as I said earlier is like learning to play the piano by listening to recorded instructions. In my experience, such an endeavor usually ultimately fails; the person gets discouraged and usually gives up. To learn the piano, you usually need instruction from someone who plays the piano and the more accomplished the player the better. You want to learn the piano from someone who plays it everyday, who is excited about it, and whose expertise is obvious. Imagine learning the piano from someone who does not play it, who gives you a tape on piano playing and says, take this home and learn to play the piano. The obstacles to learning to play the piano and learning to relax deeply are very similar except learning to deeply relax a painful pelvic floor is harder than playing the piano. I know because I do both.

Our instinct is to tighten against pain and not to relax with it, and yet I found that relaxing with the tension of certain kinds of pelvic pain can dissolve it. Learning to do this is a major event in someone's life because it is from this place that it can become possible to break the cycle of pain, anxiety, and tension and allow the sore and irritated tissue in the pelvic floor to heal.

There may be some unusual individuals who can deeply relax on a consistent basis by simply using recorded instructions and I applaud them and wish them well. The reason I do not have any faith in this is that to relax a painful pelvic floor and maintain a relaxed pelvic floor over time, (and not everybody can learn how to do this) requires guidance and instruction with regard to many issues. Examples of the issues that must be addressed are; what to do with the pain during relaxation, how to not add tension the tension of 'trying' to relax tension, when to use breathing to focus distracted mind and when to cease the breathing technique, what to do when emotions arise that the tension in the pelvic floor is suppressing, how to accept the resistance to accepting the tension, what it means to rest while there is discomfort, what to do when a plateau is reached and tension doesn't reduce, what to do when symptoms abate during relaxation and then resume quickly afterward, how to relax in the office or on the bus as well as other issues. I have seen many patients distort what to me are clear instructions I have given them and become frustrated in their practice of relaxation. Repetitive and ongoing instruction and correction is essential. A relaxation tape usually addresses none of this and the successful resolution of these issues makes the difference between success and failure.

To learn to relax the pelvic floor, especially in the presence of pain, is an enigma and the method to do this is anti-intuitive. Furthermore, it is often frightening for someone with pelvic pain to sit still with their pain and their thoughts without someone guiding and supporting them in doing so. In my experience, people avoid the kind of relaxation required to relax a tight and painful pelvis if there is no guidance and support. Recorded tapes eventually wind up on the shelf.

Few professionals whom I have offered to train in teaching this method have been interested. I think that the reason is that they were not motivated, like my pain motivated me, to spend the time to learn to do the relaxation themselves. The best teachers of this method are turning out to be the patients I have trained who are doing well themselves and use the relaxation on a daily basis.

When our treatment is effective, it can reduce symptoms very quickly in some individuals, or more typically can take between three months and two years for much of the effect of treatment to occur. We are encouraged when even small gains are seen that are associated with the use of our protocol. Small and sporadic gains are typical in the beginning of the treatment of someone who later has large and substantial reductions in symptoms. Patience and management of expectations are important for our patients. We believe that most pelvic pain did not occur overnight (although in some cases, it appears to have come on suddenly) and does not abate or disappear quickly.

CHAPTER 6

MYOFASCIAL/TRIGGER POINT RELEASE INSIDE AND OUTSIDE THE PELVIS

Rehabilitating the chronically tense tissues inside the pelvic floor

When our physical therapists do *Myofascial/Trigger Point Release* outside and inside the pelvis, they are coaxing the tissues that have become used to being contracted and painful into being comfortable, out of pain, and able to relax. We do this in a direct, hands-on way communicating to the contracted tissue through trigger point release, stretch, skin rolling and other self treatment methods inside and outside the pelvic floor that it is okay to be relaxed and out of pain.

Myofascial/Trigger Point Release has the aim of rehabilitating the tissues in and around the pelvic floor. Furthermore, we want to help strengthen weakened muscles, restore the capacity of those muscles to relax, restore the competence of the blood vessels that serve this area to soften the muscles around the nerves and to re-introduce the experience of lengthening, loosening, and quieting down in and around the pelvic floor.

The necessity of repetitive treatment

The average number of treatments for *Myofascial/Trigger Point Release* is between 10 and 40 sessions. The reason why so many treatments are necessary is that by repeatedly stretching, lengthening, and softening the pelvic tissue with manual techniques, we override its tendency to be shortened and contracted.

It is as if the *Myofascial/Trigger Point Release* therapist is saying to the tissue, "*I know you are distressed. I know you are hurting. I know you are tense and contracted. I am going to release you to give you room to breathe, to be nourished and to rest. At first it is going to hurt because you are used to being tense and contracted, so any stretching that I do to you will feel uncomfortable and unknown. You are used to being uncomfortable and so any sense of comfort, while feeling good, may not feel like 'home' to you. With my fingers I remind you over and over again that it is okay to lengthen and soften and relax. I am going to press on the knotted trigger points in you and stretch you regularly so that the lengthened state becomes normal for you. As I do this, the stretching will be both painful and paradoxically may also feel good. Patients sometimes say the pain during treatment 'hurts so well'. I am your friend and want the best for you. I know that when you learn that it is okay to be out of pain, you will want to stay out of pain. I want you to feel safe being at home. Let's work together.*"

What to expect in a Myofascial/Trigger Point Release session

When you first come into the office of the physician or therapist who will do *Myofascial/Trigger Point Release,* they will examine you externally, look at your posture, and feel and evaluate all of the muscles that relate to your pelvic floor. They will determine the strength of these muscles and whether there are trigger points or tender knots in them. They will press on trigger points that may refer pain into the areas where you are symptomatic.

The external examination first assesses muscles of the trunk and lower abdomen, looking for acute trigger points that may refer symptoms to the pelvic region. The internal examination is done through the rectum in men, and either through the vagina or the rectum or both in women. Before we do an internal examination, we will review the anatomy of your pelvic muscles. We will point out how our finger will enter inside and what we will be doing inside as we feel for trigger points and areas of soft tissue restriction.

We will be clear that in order to evaluate how your muscles are related to your pain and dysfunction, we will have to press on areas that likely will be painful. We will tell you that if the pain becomes too intense, that you are in control of the session and all you need to do is tell us to stop if you want us to stop, or slow down and lighten up if you want us to slow down or reduce the pressure we are exerting. We find that our initial examination appears to be less stressful and less painful when our patients know what to expect.

Our description of the first sessions of *Myofascial/Trigger Point Release* may sound formidable. While we can't completely assuage the anxieties of our patients who have never experienced it, it is safe to say that the *Myofascial/Trigger Point Release* is nothing to be nervous about. At worst, it is likened to going to the dentist's office.

Both the examination and the treatment of the inside of the pelvic floor in the male patient are usually done while he is lying in the prone position (on his stomach) with pillows under his pelvis. Occasionally men will be examined and treated in the lithotomy position (on the back with knees bent and open). Women can be examined prone, on their side, or on their back, depending on the area of the pelvic floor that needs to be reached.

We reach the inside of the pelvis with a gloved finger, liberally lubricated to avoid chafing or irritating the pelvic tissue. We begin by entering the rectum in men and examining the *sphincter ani* (the rings of muscle at the opening of the rectum), and then moving to the *coccygeus muscle* and then moving to the back, middle and front of the *levator ani muscles.*

We carefully check the *obturator internus muscle* because of its relationship to the *pudendal nerve*, which runs through the pelvis and *posterior ligaments*—compression or pinching of this nerve is sometimes the source of pain in certain patients.

We usually examine the left side of the body using the right hand, and the right side of the body using the left hand. Using the finger as the instrument of treatment requires that the therapist is in a certain position to gain maximum strength in palpating and stretching the trigger points. Using the hand that is opposite the side of the patient's pelvic floor (right hand to left pelvic floor, and left hand to the right pelvic floor) affords maximum leverage and extension inside.

In our digital rectal examination of male patients, we work with the trigger points that are often found in the insertions of the muscles into the pelvis around the prostate. As we assess and work with the trigger points on the edge of the prostate we move into the anterior, then middle, then *posterior levator ani muscles,* and then move to the *piriformis* and *coccygeus muscles*. In a 90-degree position (with the finger perpendicular), we move to the side-wall of the pelvis to assess the *obturator muscles.*

A session generally starts outside the pelvis, including the *lower abdominal and oblique muscles* with the trigger points found, as it helps prepare the patient for internal work. The treatment of the external muscles illustrated later in this chapter consists of trigger point release, stretching of restricted soft tissue, followed by heat and instructions for the home stretching program if they are applicable. We examine and treat the following muscles; *abdominals, psoas, quadratus, lumborum, gluteals, piriformis, abductors, pectineus, and levators.* We work on these muscles with the patient lying in different postures to facilitate lengthening of the tissue and to deactivate trigger points during this phase of treatment. We demonstrate and describe that this is what we need to do with the internal muscles so that the patient is fully informed.

In our examination we use a four point system to identify the levels of pain and tenderness of the trigger points (o = no pain, 1+ = mild pain, 2+ = moderate pain, 3+ = severe pain). When trigger points are pressed, very often the pressure will prompt someone to jump. This is called "the jump sign" and corroborates the existence of a trigger point. When there is a jump response, or a very tender area, we indicate that by using the designation 3+.

Kinds of techniques used inside the pelvic floor

The only way we can control what we do inside the pelvic floor is with the sensitivity of the finger. In a sense assessing and treating the pelvic floor is like using brail. We can't see what we are doing and must rely on the information coming through the sensitivity of a gloved finger.

We use several techniques under these conditions. The most common is called "the pressure/release technique." It has been called the technique of "ischemic compression." You will understand this method if you apply pressure to the back of your left hand with your right index finger. You will notice that when you press on the back of your hand and then release it, that a little white spot is temporarily created where the blood was pushed out by the finger pressure. This is what we do inside the pelvic floor.

We feel for the typical "taut band," characteristic of the trigger point, and apply pressure to it to help reduce and lengthen it. We hold this pressure for 30-90 seconds, while always staying in communication with our patient about their level of discomfort. Pressing on trigger points like this, especially at first, can be quite uncomfortable. The tolerance a patient has for pressure release of trigger points is improved to the extent to which they feel they can control the duration and intensity of the pressure. We proceed systematically throughout the pelvic floor to the trigger points we have identified, applying this pressure/release technique.

We sometimes use another technique developed by George Thiele in the 1940's. His method involves a sweeping motion, stroking the length of the muscle. We sometimes stroke or apply pressure to a trigger point until we feel it lengthen and soften. At that point we ask the patient to tighten the muscle up while we press against it. Then we ask the patient to relax and let go of the tightening. This method helps lengthen and soften certain rigid pelvic muscles.

After a number of treatments, which vary from patient to patient, the sensitivity of the external and internal trigger points tends to diminish, and we are left with certain internal trigger points. Sessions that last one hour at the beginning of therapy can then be reduced to 20 or 30 minutes as the rehabilitation of the pelvic muscles occurs.

Sometimes we ask patients to take hot baths before a *Myofascial/Trigger Point Release* treatment session as a way of helping loosen muscles that are tight and constricted. We often give patients warm compresses or ask them to take a warm bath after treatment as well.

Flare-ups from treatment

We tell patients that they will have flare-ups throughout treatment. This is a very important communication, because if the patient's expectation is that there will be a steady and unflagging improvement in symptoms, the flare-up after treatment can feel like a defeat and an invalidation.

Flare-ups are inevitable and frequent. In deactivating painful trigger points and stretching tissue that has been shortened for many years, it is usually not possible to avoid pain and flare-ups. It is as if the tissue is saying, *"I am not used to being so lengthened and softened. I have been tight and rigid for a long time and you are breaking my grip and holding. That hurts."* The flare-up can be seen as a good thing because it tends to corroborate our diagnosis and it tells us that we are in the right place. As the *Myofascial/Trigger Point Release* work continues, pain and discomfort associated with it tends to diminish.

Frequency of treatment

There does not seem to be a formula determining the minimum or maximum number of treatments required to achieve success with *Myofascial/Trigger Point Release.* Some patients respond immediately and require only minimal rehabilitation of the internal pelvic musculature coordinated with good *Paradoxical Relaxation* skills. Some patients need extensive treatments because of a tendency to return to a baseline tension level. We usually do not do less than ten treatments with a patient. Some patients have done 40-50 sessions as a maximum number. Some people respond quickly with 80-100% relief, while others respond much more slowly at first with 20-30% relief, even after the 12th or 13th visit. When there is *some* improvement there is more likelihood of continued improvement.

Myofascial/Trigger Point Release and the release of emotions

Sometimes during the course of internal *Myofascial/Trigger Point Release* deep emotions related to the tightness in the pelvis arise. These emotions are often related to feelings that have been suppressed in relationship to some kind of trauma or significant emotional event. Crying, fear, and anger sometimes arise and these can occur at home or in the office.

It is important to understand that the release of these emotions (they don't always occur) is part of the resolution of the condition being treated. It should be looked upon positively. Understanding that the expression of these emotions is a good thing, the partner or therapist present with the patient can be most helpful by just allowing the reaction in a caring and open way. There is nothing to be alarmed about when these emotions arise. People usually feel a sense of relief after these experiences. Sometimes it is appropriate to explore these emotions in psychotherapy as a way of resolving them.

Preparation for Myofascial/Trigger Point Release

The *Myofascial/Trigger Point Release* sessions are best regarded as special times that need to be protected from the demands of the outside world. It is for this reason that we suggest the patient come to the *Myofascial/ Trigger Point Release* treatment in a relaxed way and not running out of the car, late for the appointment because they were caught in traffic. Furthermore, it is often not prudent to schedule a demanding or stressful event after treatment. If possible, go home, bathe, rest, do a relaxation session focusing on feeling and accepting the sensations that are present in you as the result of the *Myofascial/Trigger Point Release* work.

It works best, when possible, to either arrange for a lighter day following the *Myofascial/Trigger Point Release*, or at least to keep in mind that you might be in a more vulnerable state the day after. This attitude is in keeping with understanding that the nature of treatment is aimed at making a profound change, which requires all of your support and respect.

Training the spouse or partner to do Myofascial/Trigger Point Release

When possible, we like to train the spouse or partner of the patient to do the internal and external *Myofascial/Trigger Point Release*. These techniques can be learned with competent instruction. Patients often do well having the myofascial release done by a sincerely willing partner.

Training the partner in *Myofascial/Trigger Point Release* is particularly important when a patient lives far away and there is no professional near by trained in our methodology. In these cases, the partner can do the internal stretching of trigger points at home to facilitate the pelvic floor rehabilitation which is vital to our treatment.

Explaining the Details of Physical Therapy Used in The Stanford Protocol

There is often an understandable confusion among many who wish to follow our protocol about how to tell what useful physical therapy is and isn't and how you know if you are getting the right physical therapy when you have pelvic pain. Our perspective comes from working with many patients who have seen us at Stanford and with whom we have used the Stanford protocol over the years.

We have interviewed many patients who have seen a variety of physical therapists. We have listened carefully to the comparison of their experiences to their experiences with physical therapists we know are competent in our protocol. We have looked at the results and want to discuss these comparisons below.

In putting together a brief description of the phenomenon of myofascial restriction and trigger point activity related to the pelvic floor in this chapter, we are not suggesting that anyone use this information as a substitute for proper in-person physical therapy training nor are we suggesting that one treats oneself without proper instruction and training. Competently doing our physical therapy protocol is not mastered quickly but by a thorough understanding of the trigger point phenomenon and by experience in successfully working with *Myofascial/Trigger Point Release* in and outside of the pelvic floor. Knowing what we know now, at the release of this third edition, we believe that there are still very few physical therapists to whom we could confidently send our patients. Over the past few years we have offered training for physical therapists in our approach. The response to taking these trainings has been tepid. We hope this will change.

Physical therapy works together with Paradoxical Relaxation

We wish to reiterate that physical therapy is one part of the equation of treating a certain kind of pelvic pain. It is tempting to see an external fix like *Myofascial/Trigger Point Release* as the answer to pelvic pain. When you have pelvic pain of the kind we treat and decide to do whatever it takes to resolve it, you find out there is no quick fix but results come from committing yourself to the inside job of changing very stubborn inner habits.

The most exhaustive physical therapy done brilliantly, while essential in our protocol, cannot guarantee that the offending trigger points will behave. Consider that there are 168 hours in a week. Let us say that a person goes to see the physical therapist 2 times a week. That is quite a bit of physical therapy. In the physical therapy session, after a person takes off their clothes, gives the physical therapist a report on their week and begins the physical therapy itself, at the most there is probably 30-45 minutes of hands-on treatment. After the treatment, the tissue is stretched (although sometimes temporarily irritated in the process). That is at the most 1-1/2 hours of therapeutic treatment per week. In a good pelvic floor physical therapy session, the pelvic floor tissue has been lengthened and life has been made more livable for it.

However, after physical therapy, there are about 166 hours remaining in the week. The old habit of going 100 miles an hour in one's life and tightening up the pelvis regularly and squeezing and shortening the irritated tissue can easily and quickly undo the therapeutic impact of the physical therapy session. A physical therapy treatment that lasts less that 1% of your life cannot work if the old, symptom-provoking habits go on unabated. This is the why the ongoing regular relaxation of the pelvic floor and quieting of the nervous system with the relaxation protocol like the one we use is necessary. The resolution of the kind of pelvic pain we treat is an inside job of cooperating with the healing mechanism of the body in the short run and the long run. *Myofascial/Trigger Point Release* is an essential and necessary component but not a sufficient one by itself.

That all being said, we now address the issue of what physical therapy works for pelvic pain and what criteria there are to evaluate the physical therapy you are getting or want to get. Seeing someone who is a physical therapist and even seeing someone who holds him or herself out as a pelvic floor physical therapist offers no guarantee that our protocol will be followed. This is critical information for the patient who sees hope for his condition using our protocol and is intent on undergoing it. One can do physical therapy for pelvic pain with a physical therapist with little understanding and experience in *Myofascial/Trigger Point Release* and receive little benefit. Going to a different physical therapist who is trained, talented, and experienced can make a huge difference.

In other words the experience, understanding and intuitive talent of a physical therapist doing myofascial trigger point release can make the difference between success and failure of our protocol and the reduction or resolution of one's symptoms or not.

Let us move on to a discussion of *Myofascial/Trigger Point Release.* Doctors Travell and Simons were the originators of *Myofascial/Trigger Point Release* therapy. They published the first edition of *Myofascial Pain and Dysfunction: The Trigger Point Manual* in 1983, followed by a second edition in 1992. These books were the culmination of research that went back to 1942 when Dr. Janet Travell published her first article on myofascial pain. It is not well know that she was appointed as the White House physician during the Kennedy and Johnson administration as an expression of Kennedy's gratitude for her successful treatment of his myofascial pain that threatened to end his political career.

The concept of trigger points is relatively new to medicine. It is very new to urology. Trigger points are defined as taut bands within a muscle, either at the surface of the muscle or inside the muscle, in the belly or the attachment of the muscle. The trigger point characteristically elicits a twitch response, detectable on ultrasound or via electromyography (that measures the electrical activity in a muscle in millionths of a volt) that can be felt by a trained and sensitive practitioner while palpating the trigger point. When the trigger point is pressed there is often a 'jump' response in the patient, due to the reflexive reaction of the patient to the often exquisite tenderness of the trigger point upon palpation. Furthermore, the trigger point characteristically refers pain/sensation to the site being pressed or to a site remote from it.

A trigger point can be active or latent. An active trigger point is considered able to refer pain and recreate that pain upon palpation when the patient comes in with a complaint of pain. A latent trigger point has the capacity to be the source of pain (i.e., has the capacity to become an active one) and under certain circumstances, becomes active but generally the patient does not complain of symptoms from latent trigger points. Trigger points are latent in many people. *Often active trigger points never entirely go away with the best therapy and so the goal of both our physical therapy and Paradoxical Relaxation protocol is to manage the trigger points so that they stop being symptomatic.*

The problem that occurs when urologists are asked to consider trigger points as essential ingredients in chronic pelvic pain syndromes is the problem of a 'paradigm conflict.' Our book presents a very different paradigm from the paradigm of conventional medicine. A paradigm is a model of reality. Urologists have little or no training or understanding of the role of trigger points in pelvic pain. The connective tissue and muscles inside and outside the pelvis are the sites in which many offending trigger points are found. This tissue and the trigger points that are found there, in many pelvic pain patients, have rarely been taken seriously as a source of pain by most urologists. This concept of trigger points in urology is poorly understood and not readily accepted for reasons that we discussed earlier in our book.

The site where one feels the trigger point pain is often not the source of the pain. For this reason pelvic pain diagnosed by someone unfamiliar with the workings of trigger points is often mistaken because they are unclear that the source of much pelvic pain is not where it seems to be. In other words, pain coming from trigger points often is not coming from where you feel the pain. While doctors understand the concept of referred pain, the idea that pelvic pain felt in the groin, penis, testicles or vagina, clitoris, vulva or the perineum may indeed originate inside the pelvic floor is a not part of a urologists training, understanding or belief. Part of the difficulty that doctors have with trigger points is that they have usually received no training in the subject. Furthermore, because there is no objective, litmus paper, gold standard test for evaluating them and the only way clinically to find and treat them is through palpation, which requires training and a sensitive touch, trigger points do not exist in the reality of many doctors. This is part of the paradigm conflict.

This paradigm conflict has very real consequences to patients with pelvic pain. Recently, we received a call from a woman who had very severe rectal pain. She reported that during the course of one of her doctor's pelvic exams, he hit a spot that the woman said, "sent me through the roof." After the exam, the doctor told her that he really did not know what was going on with her, that he couldn't help her and she might simply have to live with the pain. The woman went home despondent, her pelvic floor very irritated and flared up. *The next day she woke up and her pain was almost gone. It remained so for several days.* She called up the doctor's office happily bewildered to share with the doctor what happened. She told the nurse that she thought it was related to the painful spot the doctor pressed. The nurse relayed the news about the woman to the doctor. The doctor then told the nurse to tell the patient she could massage that point herself if it helped her. The patient felt more bewildered.

What probably happened is that the doctor inadvertently pressed and temporarily released a major trigger point for the woman and the woman responded like any of our patients typically respond with some flare up and then a reduction of symptoms. The doctor, in not understanding anything about trigger point pain and treatment, essentially dismissed this event and the possibility of helping this woman. His ignorance may have had a profound effect on his patient. She remained confused even after we spoke to her.

Trigger points refer pain directly on the trigger point site or to a remote site, which means that where you feel the pain is often not where it actually is coming from. For instance, trigger points in women on the obturator internus can refer pain to the vulva, vagina, and urethra. In men, we find that tip-of-the-penis pain is often referred from trigger points in the anterior portion of the *levator ani muscle* as it attaches to the prostate. This is not obvious and is anti-intuitive. These trigger points are a good five inches from where the pain is occurring. Who would think that the source of genital pain would come from a site so far away? To complicate matters further, if you do not have long enough fingers or if you do not understand how the trigger points work in the body, you miss this connection entirely. And if you don't want to keep pressure on an internal trigger point for the length of time we know is necessary, the trigger point remains active.

The internal muscles that contain trigger points are close to each other and it takes someone who understands the internal pelvic anatomy and is experienced in feeling the muscles inside the pelvic floor, to tell them apart. You can see the location of these muscles to which I am referring in the illustrations that follow. Below are a list of the muscles in which most internal trigger points are found. The relationship between symptoms and the location of associated trigger points is described below. Some of the connections reported below have not been previously published and come from the extensive experience of our senior physical therapist Tim Sawyer.

All of the muscles, both internal and external, must be thoroughly evaluated and treated. When muscles are known to contain trigger points referring pain to an area that the patient is complaining about, they should be extra carefully examined. The therapist must be trained in identifying trigger points and able to feel for superficial and deep trigger points located in the belly and the attachments of the muscles. And it is very important that when trigger points are located, they must be held with pressure release which involves pressing on a trigger point with constant pressure, usually for a period of 60-90 seconds. When appropriate the following techniques are used:

- Voluntary contraction and release/hold-relax/contract-relax/ reciprocal inhibition
- Spray and stretch occasionally with stubborn external trigger points
- Deep tissue mobilization including striping, strumming, effleurage
- Skin rolling
- Myofascial/trigger point release
- Strain-counter-strain/ muscle energy release

Anyone who has pelvic pain of the kind we treat should know that specific trigger points in specific pelvic muscles tend to refer specific kinds of symptoms. This knowledge is critical for the physical therapist that is treating pelvic pain. For example, pain in the tip of the penis or the sense of urgency and frequency is typically created by active trigger points in the anterior (front) portion of the *levator ani muscle* as it attaches to the prostate. When the physician or physical therapist does an examination, knowledge of the relationship between symptoms and pelvic trigger points is essential to make the diagnosis of tension/ neuromuscular related pelvic pain and dysfunction. When we find relationships between trigger points and the kinds of symptoms they typically refer, as presented below, we are much more confident in our diagnosis and ability to help the patient.

The illustrations to follow indicate the internal pelvic and external pelvic floor related trigger points and the location of the pain and symptoms they typically refer. Certainly, not all patients fit all the patterns we describe here. Sometimes only one or two trigger points fit the referral pattern we describe. To reiterate, we sometimes can help people with tight and tender pelvic muscles where we find no discernable trigger points. this technique.

Internal Pelvic Floor Trigger Points and Where They Typically Refer Pain and Sensation

In working internally, we generally work with patients in the prone position with a cushion under their stomach, an innovation of the physical therapist, Tim Sawyer. The right hand is used to examine and work the left side of the pelvic floor and the left hand to work the right side of the pelvic floor. Patients tend to feel less vulnerable and more comfortable in this position and it affords the practitioner good access inside and outside the pelvic floor.

The following illustrations show trigger points in the internal pelvic muscles.

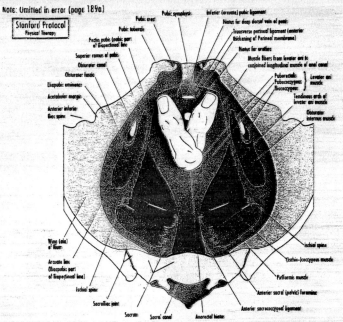

Anterior Levator Ani, Superior portion (or Puborectalis)

This is one of the most important trigger point sites in male pelvic pain and palpating high enough up and firmly enough is critical in proper treatment. Frequently this area is the site of trigger points that are responsible for the tip-of-the-penis and shaft-of-the-penis-pain. Furthermore, trigger points in this area can refer to the bladder, urethra, pressure, and fullness in the prostate.

- Most important trigger point site for male pelvic pain
- Can refer tip-of-the-penis, shaft-of-the-penis, bladder urethral pain
- Can refer pressure/fullness in prostate

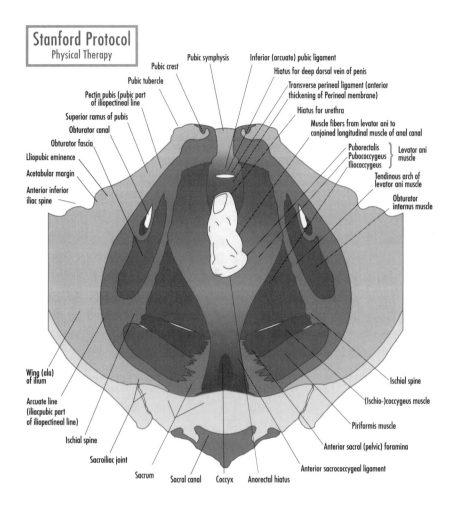

Stanford Protocol
Physical Therapy

Pubic symphysis
Pubic crest
Pubic tubercle
Pectin pubis (pubic part of iliopectineal line)
Superior ramus of pubis
Obturator canal
Obturator fascia
Lliopubic eminence
Acetabular margin
Anterior inferior iliac spine

Inferior (arcuate) pubic ligament
Hiatus for deep dorsal vein of penis
Transverse perineal ligament (anterior thickening of Perineal membrane)
Hiatus for urethra
Muscle fibers from levator ani to conjoined longitudinal muscle of anal canal
Puborectalis
Pubococcygeus } Levator ani muscle
Iliococcygeus
Tendinous arch of levator ani muscle
Obturator internus muscle

Wing (ala) of ilium
Arcuate line (iliacpubic part of iliopectineal line)
Ischial spine
Sacroiliac joint
Sacrum
Sacral canal
Coccyx
Anorectal hiatus

Ischial spine
(Ischio-)coccygeus muscle
Piriformis muscle
Anterior sacral (pelvic) foramina
Anterior sacrococcygeal ligament

Anterior Levator Ani, inferior portion

- *Can refer to perineum and base of the penis*

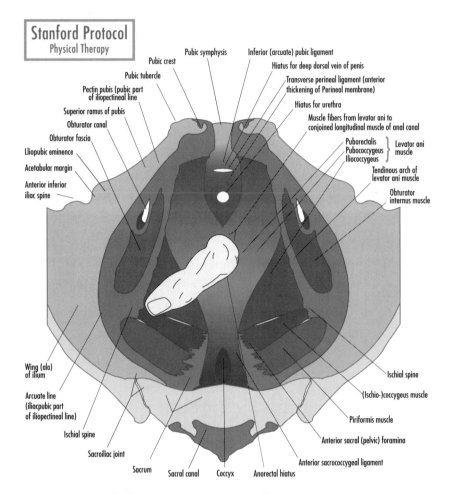

Middle Levator Ani - (Iliococcygeus)

Trigger points in the middle levator ani (iliococcygeus) typically refer lateral wall pain, perineal pain and anal sphincter pain. Trigger points can refer forward toward the anterior levators and the prostate. Trigger points here can refer discomfort associated with a sense of prostate fullness.

> • *Can refer lateral wall, perineal, anal sphincter, prostate fullness*
> *pain/discomfort referral pattern toward the anterior levators and*
> *prostate*

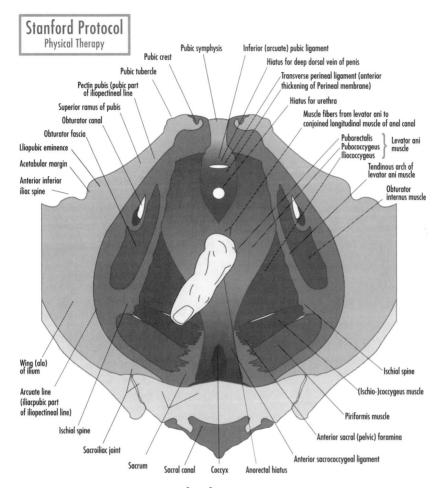

Stanford Protocol
Physical Therapy

Pubic symphysis
Pubic crest
Pubic tubercle
Pectin pubis (pubic part of iliopectineal line)
Superior ramus of pubis
Obturator canal
Obturator fascia
Iliopubic eminence
Acetabular margin
Anterior inferior iliac spine

Inferior (arcuate) pubic ligament
Hiatus for deep dorsal vein of penis
Transverse perineal ligament (anterior thickening of Perineal membrane)
Hiatus for urethra
Muscle fibers from levator ani to conjoined longitudinal muscle of anal canal
Puborectalis
Pubococcygeus } Levator ani muscle
Iliococcygeus
Tendinous arch of levator ani muscle
Obturator internus muscle

Wing (ala) of ilium
Arcuate line (iliacpubic part of iliopectineal line)
Ischial spine
Sacroiliac joint
Sacrum
Sacral canal
Coccyx
Anorectal hiatus

Ischial spine
(Ischio-)coccygeus muscle
Piriformis muscle
Anterior sacral (pelvic) foramina
Anterior sacrococcygeal ligament

Coccygeus/Ischio-coccygeus

Trigger points in this muscle typically refers pain and pressure associated with the sense of have a golf-ball-in-the-rectum, pain to the coccyx and gluteus maximus. Pre or post bowel movement pain is often associated with the sense of having a full bowel.

- **Can refer symptoms** *to coccygeus, coccyx, gluteus maximus, pre or post bowel movement pain/full bowel sensation and discomfort*

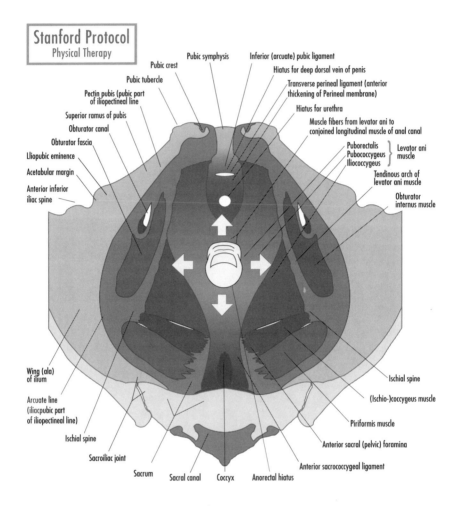

Sphincter Ani

Trigger points in this area may cause anal pain in the anal sphinter itself as well as pain going toward the front and back part of the anal sphincter. Treatment is done by gently stretching the sphincter upward in the 12 o'clock position, sideways in the 3 o'clock position, downward to the 6 o'clock position and sideways toward the 9 o'clock position.

- *Can refer pain in the anal sphincter itself as well as radiating to the front and back from the sphincter*

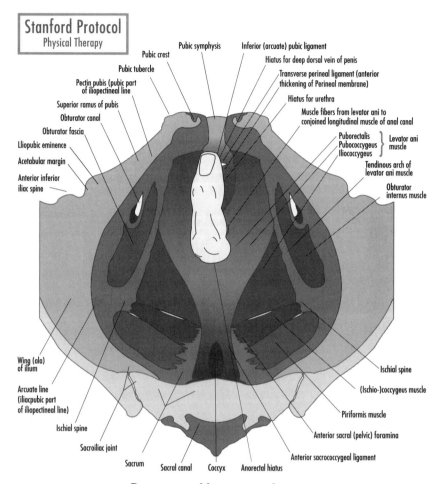

Stanford Protocol
Physical Therapy

Pubic symphysis
Pubic crest
Pubic tubercle
Pectin pubis (pubic part of iliopectineal line)
Superior ramus of pubis
Obturator canal
Obturator fascia
Lliopubic eminence
Acetabular margin
Anterior inferior iliac spine

Inferior (arcuate) pubic ligament
Hiatus for deep dorsal vein of penis
Transverse perineal ligament (anterior thickening of Perineal membrane)
Hiatus for urethra
Muscle fibers from levator ani to conjoined longitudinal muscle of anal canal
Puborectalis
Pubococcygeus } Levator ani muscle
Iliococcygeus
Tendinous arch of levator ani muscle
Obturator internus muscle

Wing (ala) of ilium
Arcuate line (iliacpubic part of iliopectineal line)
Ischial spine
Sacroiliac joint
Sacrum
Sacral canal
Coccyx
Anorectal hiatus

Ischial spine
(Ischio-)coccygeus muscle
Piriformis muscle
Anterior sacral (pelvic) foramina
Anterior sacrococcygeal ligament

Prostate Massage Area

- *Traditionally urologists massage the prostate to extract prostatic fluid in order to examine it under the microscope or to drain the prostate of inflammation or infection. The massage of the prostate in the Stanford Protocol is not done for this purpose. We massage the prostate when the physician specifically prescribes this massage or we do it to stretch the associated connective tissue. While some physicians do prostate massage vigorously or roughly, we do not. Especially if the prostate is tender, we are very gentle at first and our purpose is to desensitize the sensitivity of the prostate so that with repeated ongoing massage over a period of a number of massages, the prostate becomes less painful. Our method of prostate massage is as follows. We locate the prostate and do lateral sweeps from outside to inside when the finger is on one side (lateral to medial) of the prostate. And then from the other side with same hand, we do lateral to medial (outside to inside) sweeps ...always going from the outside to the center of the prostate. We then go from top to the bottom (superior to inferior). If the prostate is excrutiatingly painful, we are particularly gentle. The duration of the entire massage is approximately one minute.*

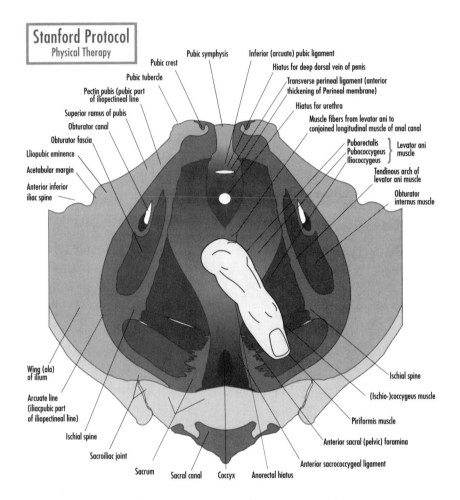

Stanford Protocol
Physical Therapy

Pubic symphysis
Pubic crest
Pubic tubercle
Pectin pubis (pubic part of iliopectineal line)
Superior ramus of pubis
Obturator canal
Obturator fascia
Iliopubic eminence
Acetabular margin
Anterior inferior iliac spine

Inferior (arcuate) pubic ligament
Hiatus for deep dorsal vein of penis
Transverse perineal ligament (anterior thickening of Perineal membrane)
Hiatus for urethra
Muscle fibers from levator ani to conjoined longitudinal muscle of anal canal
Puborectalis
Pubococcygeus
Iliococcygeus
Levator ani muscle
Tendinous arch of levator ani muscle
Obturator internus muscle

Wing (ala) of ilium
Arcuate line (iliacpubic part of iliopectineal line)
Ischial spine
Sacroiliac joint

Sacrum   Sacral canal   Coccyx   Anorectal hiatus

Ischial spine
(Ischio-)coccygeus muscle
Piriformis muscle
Anterior sacral (pelvic) foramina
Anterior sacrococcygeal ligament

Piriformis (internally accessed)

Trigger points here can refer to the sacroiliac joint, the hip girdle and hamstrings. Patients can feel increased pain at the palpation site.

- *Can refer to sacroiliac joint, hip girdle, hamstrings and increased pain at palpation site*

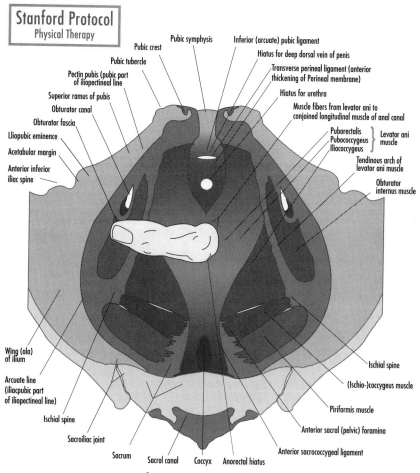

Obturator Internus

Trigger points in the obturator can refer pain to the perineum, outward toward hip, to the whole pelvic floor both anteriorly and posteriorly. The obturator is intimate with the pudendal nerve and can refer a dull ache and burning in the pelvic floor on the side that it is being palpated. Trigger points in the obturator can refer the golf-ball-in-the-rectum feeling, symptoms to the coccyx, hamstrings and posterior thigh. In women, trigger points in the obturator can refer to the urethra, the vagina, and specifically the vulva and is a very important point in the treatment of vulvar pain.

- *Can refer dull ache on the side palpated, golf-ball-in-the-rectum sensation, coccyx, hamstrings, posterior thigh, urethra, vagina, vulva (important in vulvodynia)*

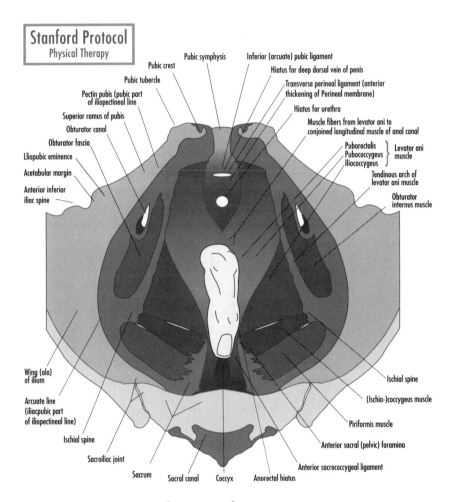

Stanford Protocol
Physical Therapy

Pubic symphysis

Pubic crest

Inferior (arcuate) pubic ligament

Pubic tubercle

Hiatus for deep dorsal vein of penis

Pectin pubis (pubic part of iliopectineal line)

Transverse perineal ligament (anterior thickening of Perineal membrane)

Superior ramus of pubis

Hiatus for urethra

Obturator canal

Muscle fibers from levator ani to conjoined longitudinal muscle of anal canal

Obturator fascia

Puborectalis
Pubococcygeus
Iliococcygeus } Levator ani muscle

Lliopubic eminence

Acetabular margin

Tendinous arch of levator ani muscle

Anterior inferior iliac spine

Obturator internus muscle

Wing (ala) of ilium

Ischial spine

Arcuate line (iliacpubic part of iliopectineal line)

(Ischio-)coccygeus muscle

Ischial spine

Piriformis muscle

Sacroiliac joint

Anterior sacral (pelvic) foramina

Anterior sacrococcygeal ligament

Sacrum

Sacral canal

Coccyx

Anorectal hiatus

Palpating the coccyx

This is a bony palpation. In treating pelvic pain, if the coccyx is immobile, it can be a factor that perpetuates trigger points that cause pelvic pain.

> • *An immobile coccyx can perpetuate pelvic pain*

External Pelvic Floor Trigger Points and Where They Typically Refer Pain and Sensation

External trigger points can be as important in perpetuating a pain cycle as internal trigger points. For example we treated a man for whom significant groin pain came from his *quadratus lumborum muscle,* located on the side of the body. Again, this trigger point was relatively far away from where the pain was felt. When this trigger point was treated, the man experienced tremendous relief. Every doctor that this man saw in the years he suffered with this trigger point missed this. We have treated people who have had abdominal trigger points that refer excruciating pain into the pelvis.

To the therapist experienced in *Myofascial/Trigger Point Release,* the patient's symptoms, as well as the physical examination give the essential clues as to the location of the trigger points. We are grateful to Dr. David Simons, coauthor of *Myofascial Pain and Dysfunction: The Trigger Point Manual*,* and his publisher for allowing us to use the original drawings in his book. We have taken the liberty of adding a pointing finger on each drawing. The tip of the pointing finger marks the location of the trigger point likely to be causing the pain patterns illustrated in the shaded areas.

The following illustrations show trigger points in the external muscles that can contribute to pelvic pain.

* The identification under each drawing of external trigger points related to pelvic pain herein provides easy reference to the volume number and figure where the drawing originated in *Myofascial Pain and Dysfunction: The Trigger Point Manual,* 2nd edition by Janet G. Travell and David G. Simons, published copyright held by Lippincott Williams & Wilkins, (October 1, 1998). Original drawings by Barbara Abeloff. Proofreading and editing by Lois S. Simons. Copyright 1989, Lippincott Williams & Wilkins.

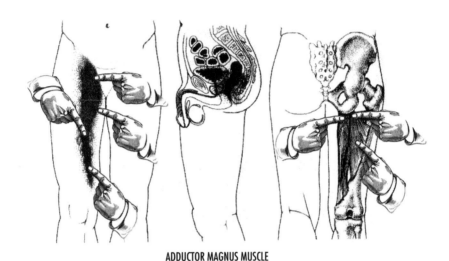

Stanford Protocol
Physical Therapy

ADDUCTOR MAGNUS MUSCLE
v.2 Fig. 15.2

Pain felt in shaded area
Finger tip locates trigger point

ADDUCTOR MAGNUS

- *This muscle is missed by many clinicians*
- *The adductor magnus is a critical muscle to check for trigger points which can refer pain throughout the pelvic floor including perineum, bladder and prostate*
- *When trigger points continue to be active internally, the culprit may be unresolved trigger points in the adductor magnus*
- *Trigger points in the adductor magnus can refer the sensation of having a golf ball in the rectum*

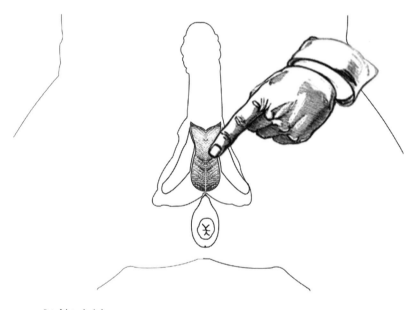

Pain felt in shaded area
Finger tip locates trigger point

BULBOSPONGIOSIS AND ISCHIOCAVERNOSIS

- Trigger points in the bulbospongiosis and ischiocavernosis can refer pain and sensation *to the base of the penis and the perineum*

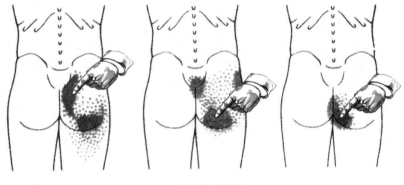

GLUTEUS MAXIMUS
v.2 Fig. 7.1

Pain felt in shaded area
Finger tip locates trigger point

GLUTEUS (MAXIMUS)

- *Trigger points in the gluteus maximus can refer pain and sensation into the hip buttocks, tailbone, sacrum and hamstrings*

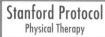

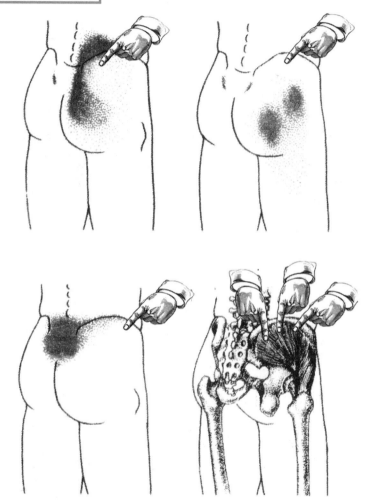

Pain felt in shaded area
Finger tip locates trigger point

GLUTEUS MEDIUS
v.2 Fig. 8.1

GLUTEUS (MEDIUS)

- *Trigger points in the gluteus medius can refer pain and sensation around the buttocks, hip girdle and down the leg as well as into the testicles*

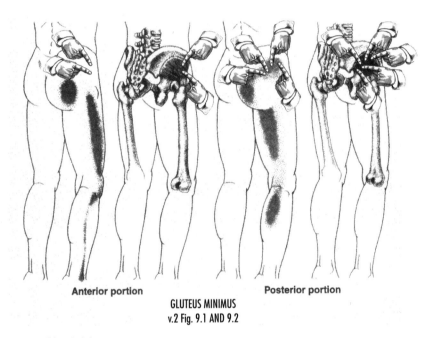

Anterior portion   **Posterior portion**

GLUTEUS MINIMUS
v.2 Fig. 9.1 AND 9.2

Pain felt in shaded area
Finger tip locates trigger point

GLUTEUS (MINIMUS)

- *Trigger points in the gluteus minimus can refer pain and sensation down the leg and sometimes into the testicles*

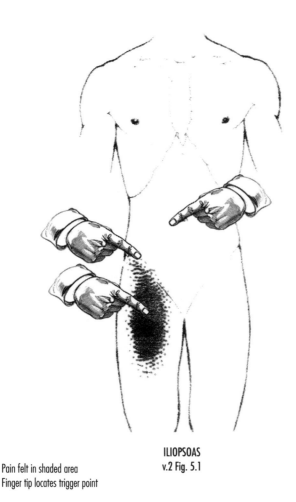

Pain felt in shaded area
Finger tip locates trigger point

ILIOPSOAS
v.2 Fig. 5.1

ILIOPSOAS

- *Trigger points in the iliopsoas can refer pain to the groin, anterior (front part) thigh and low back*

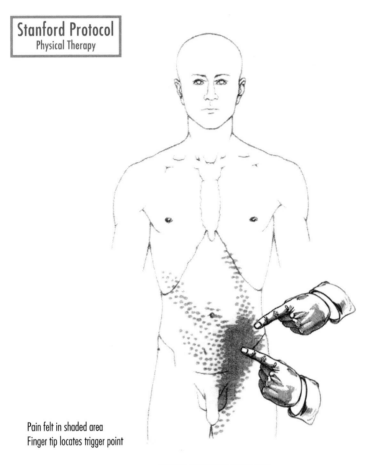

Pain felt in shaded area
Finger tip locates trigger point

LATERAL ABDOMINALS OBLIQUE
V.1 Fig. 49.1

LATERAL ABDOMINALS OBLIQUE

- *Trigger points in the lateral abdominals can refer pain to the whole stomach, up into the ribs, down the groin and into the testicles... this is an important source of testicular pain*

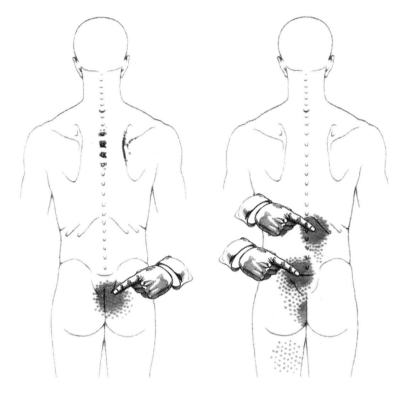

MULTIFIDI
v.1 Fig. 48.2

Pain felt in shaded area
Finger tip locates trigger point

PARASPINALS and MULTIFIDI

- *Trigger points in the paraspinals tend to refer pain and sensation into the low back however this is pain that doesn't tend to fan out but is tightly contained in a specific area*

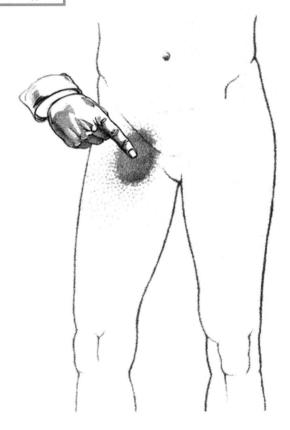

Stanford Protocol
Physical Therapy

PECTINEUS
v.2 Fig. 13.1

Pain felt in shaded area
Finger tip locates trigger point

PECTINEUS

- *Trigger points in the pectineus can refer pain and sensation to the groin... this is a major trigger point for groin pain*

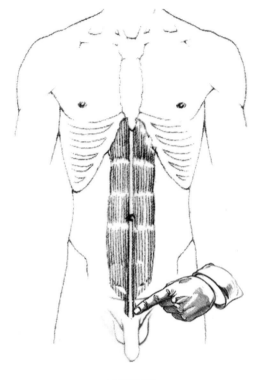

PYRAMIDALIS
v.2 Fig. 13.1

Pain felt in shaded area
Finger tip locates trigger point

PYRAMIDALIS

- *The pyramidalis is not present in some individuals but when it is present and has trigger points, they can refer pain and sensation to the bladder, pubic bone and urethra*

Modern medicine can be likened to Christianity and schools of thought in medicine to the different denominations like the Baptists, Unitarians, and Episcopalians. In the world of physical therapy, there are different churches or schools of thought about how, for instance, you do *Myofascial/Trigger Point Release.* Our protocol closely follows the methods of Travell and Simons. Many patients that we have seen have been treated previously by physical therapists using different methods. They have shared their experiences and compared them to our protocol and the others they have used. *We are convinced that the methodology we use is by far the most effective.*

Here are some important points about the Stanford Protocol for physical therapy of the pelvic floor. If the trigger point is not palpated vigorously and specifically enough, the trigger point can simply resist deactivation. Yet there is danger of injuring the tissue if the pressure is inappropriately vigorous. Experience and talent in feeling the tissue and sensing how much to palpate is imperative. Physical therapists that are not experienced in dealing specifically with pelvic pain can err in several ways—most importantly, they do not find the trigger point, and they are not vigorous enough in palpating when the trigger point is found, or they do not use pressure release on the trigger points for 60-90 seconds.

Our general rule of thumb is that the trigger point should be pressed for 60-90 seconds. This is no small feat especially when a physical therapist with delicate hands is working on a muscle inside the pelvic floor of a large and strong man or woman. A large stress is put on the physical therapist's finger in every *Myofascial/Trigger Point Release* session and the therapist's finger is prone to injury unless the finger is used properly and the therapist is endowed with a certain level of strength and a certain kind of finger. Doing *Myofascial/Trigger Point Release* therapy can put your fingers at risk of injury and it is why some physical therapists choose to not or are not able to follow our protocol.

Flare-up of symptoms is common especially after the first number of *Myofascial/Trigger Point Release* sessions. These flare ups usually abate as treatment continues although they can recur in times of a flare-up.

Without their knowledge, I have seen some inexperienced therapists back off from treatment after a patient's flare-up out of fear that they did something wrong. This concern is immediately gotten across to patients who become concerned that they are going down the wrong road. Doubt about physical therapy and the whole course of treatment arises and it is not uncommon for patients to stop treatment. This is all because the therapist did not have enough training and experience to see the big picture of treatment and the common occurrence of flare-ups after treatment.

When people do trigger point release it is best, when possible, to not immediately go back into a situation of demand and tension. If you think about the physical therapy that we do as stretching and lengthening of contracted tissue that can allow it to rest and heal, taking time after a therapy session to remain quiet and rest the pelvic floor is important. A tightened pelvic floor is usually the physical expression of a psychologically defended state and releasing the pelvic tissues can trigger emotional release and psychological insight during and/or after the physical therapy session. In our view, both the therapist and patient need to be aware of this possibility and regard such reactions as positive signs of healing. Abreactions should be allowed and not suppressed or denied.

The management of expectations in *Myofascial/Trigger Point Release* is essential and both patient and therapist must clearly understand that flare-ups are common and to be expected and progress often occurs over the period of many months. Often treatment can feel like three steps ahead and two steps back for quite a while. The idea that there should be a quick fix, and that the therapist is responsible for making it all happen often results in the failure of treatment.

There can be multiple trigger points either inside or outside the pelvic floor that refer to the same area of pain and if not all of them are treated, then the pain can persist. There is sometimes a very perplexing network of trigger points that are involved in pelvic pain to the inexperienced *Myofascial/Trigger Point Release* therapist. At this time there are few physical therapists that we refer patients to who we believe are competent in our protocol. If any inexperienced therapist is motivated to learn and the patient is willing to be patient with the therapist, a therapist new to this work can learn it. Seeing someone with little experience whose work is not being supervised by someone trained and experienced can result in disappointment and abandonment of the protocol.

We have defined what we include in our protocol and what we do not. A summary is provided.

- The emphasis of our physical therapy work with pelvic pain is on trigger point release. We consider a thorough examination of possible interior and exterior trigger points to be essential in our protocol. Our protocol is most promising when we can find internal or external trigger points that tend to recreate a patient's symptoms. It should be said that while we have the most consistent success with people in whom we can find trigger points that recreate their symptoms, sometimes we have helped people with no clear trigger points but with a much contracted pelvic floor.

- At this point, as a rule we do not use pelvic floor biofeedback therapeutically in which an anal probe is inserted and patients are asked to do EMG–monitored Kegel exercises. Also, we consider unremarkable pelvic floor biofeedback readings a poor measure of what is going on in the pelvic floor or whether our protocol is indicated. We have written about these subjects elsewhere in this book.

- Generally, we do not use electrical stimulation either at the office or for home treatment.

- Reiterating, the physical therapy emphasis for pelvic pain is on trigger point release. If postural and/or mechanical factors appear related to the pelvic pain, we refer the patient back to a physical therapist in their home area and reserve the often-precious time we have with them for trigger point release. In looking at the results of physical therapy of our patients, we have not been impressed with physical therapy for pelvic pain emphasizing posture and alignment. We know that there are physical therapists who will disagree with us.

- *Skin rolling or connective tissue massage* can be a very important self help tool which many of our patients are encouraged to use.

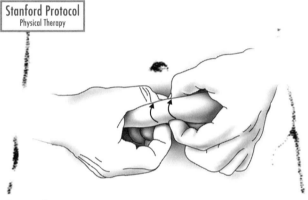

Skin Rolling

We sometimes recommend skin rolling or connective tissue massage. This method is explained below, although it is difficult to explain how to do skin rolling. It is not simply a pinching of the skin and rolling it in place but rolling the skin while moving the roll of skin downward just as a wave moves from off shore to the shore. Skin rolling is rolling the skin down or up in a moving wave. The point is that in skin rolling, you roll the skin downward, sideways or vertically but the skin roll isn't stationary-- it moves. In other words you alternately walk the fingers along the skin by continuously pushing down with the thumb and up with the index and third finger and thereby move downward, rolling the skin as the skin rolls moves downward just as a wave moves from off shore to the shore.

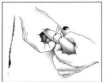
Diagonal Left

Diagonal Right

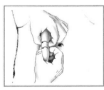
Vertical

- We encourage patients to do home trigger point release using a *Theracane*, a tennis ball and/or knobber.

- We only do prostate massage when prescribed by a physician and when the prostate is tender. It is not done routinely. From our perspective, the purpose of prostate massage is for stretching the associated connective tissue especially where it attaches to the prostate, and is not done for prostatic fluid drainage.

- While we appreciate the efficacy of Feldenkrais, craniosacral manipulation, the Alexander method, internal Thiele massage and other modalities for many kinds of problems, we generally do not use or recommend these methods for the pelvic pain we treat.

- Before and after treatment, we use gentle, moderate or deep effleurage or Swedish type massage on the external areas (gluteals, back, leg and stomach).

- Our physical therapy protocol is based on the knowledge that multiple trigger points can refer to one place and each trigger point must be evaluated and treated.

- We use pressure release of trigger points applying pressure for 60 to 90 seconds.

- We encourage patients to self-treat both internally and externally after proper supervision.

- When possible and with the patient's permission, we train the individual's partner to do our method of *Myofascial/Trigger Point Release.*

- We believe that the success of a patient, appropriate for our protocol, depends on regularly doing the home practices that we prescribe. We do not advise taking up these activities unless one is properly supervised.

The muscles of the pelvic floor are easily contracted but stretching them in the way that you can stretch your shoulders or arms is not so easily accomplished. However, they can be stretched to some degree. We consider it essential to train patients in relevant stretches. They include:

- Adductor/pectineus posture
- Lateral rotators and piriformis posture
- Cobra posture
- Pelvic tilt posture
- Knee pull posture
- Iliopsoas posture
- Quatratus lumborum posture
- Squat posture
- Adductor posture

We sometimes deem it appropriate to train the patient in the use of a self-administered myofascial/trigger point wand. We are inclined to use this especially when there is no physical therapist available near the patient's home. We are still in the experimental stage using this kind of wand.

We hope that this discussion helps to shed some light on the physical therapy that we recommend. The physical therapy discussed here is what we have seen be most helpful in alleviating the pelvic pain and symptoms we treat.

Home stretching program

We ask patients to do certain stretches several times a day throughout the week. These stretches include a stretch of the *psoas muscle,* stretching of the abdomen (which can be thought of as a trunk extension), a partial cobra stretch; a side bend stretch and sometimes pressing a tennis ball against a wall to deal with trigger points and tightness in the *quadratus lumborum.*

Stretches are also done with *adductor and pectineus muscles*. We educate our patients in doing diaphragmatic breathing while doing these stretches. When possible, we encourage patients to take a hot bath before stretching.

Home Stretches

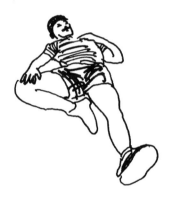

1.   Stretching the adductors (pectineus)

This stretch is done while lying down on a firm surface and first bending one knee while the other unbent leg is resting on the floor. The hand on the same side as the bent knee is placed on the inside of the knee and then slowly pushes the bent knee outward toward the floor. The bent knee is held down toward the floor by the hand for between 15 to 30 seconds and then return the bent leg is returned to the upright position or slide leg down to rest on the floor. This is repeated with the other leg. This is done 3 times or as needed during the day.

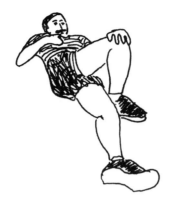

2. Stretching the lateral rotators and the piriformis

This stretch is done lying down on a firm surface and like stretch #1, one knee is bent while the other leg is resting unbent on the floor. The hand that is opposite the bent knee is placed on the outside of the bent knee and pulled down toward the floor as illustrated in picture. The stretch is held for 15 to 30 seconds. This stretch is repeated three times and done as needed during the day.

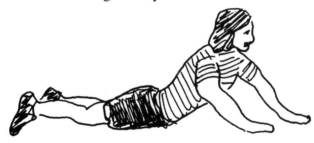

3. The Cobra

This is a well known yoga stretch and is done lying stomach down while slowly pushing upper body upward by straightening the arms and bending back the lower back. This is held for 15-30 seconds. For those with low back pain, this can be a partial cobra with the arms partially extended rather than fully extended. This stretch is repeated three times and done as needed during the day.

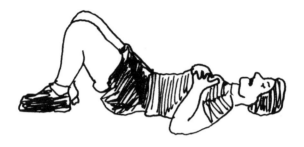

4.   Pelvic tilt

This stretch is done on a firm surface, face up with both knees bent. The abdomen and buttocks are tightened with the result of rocking the pelvis and putting the lower back flat against the floor. The lower back is held for 5-10 seconds against the floor and then rested. This is done 3 times and done as needed during the day.

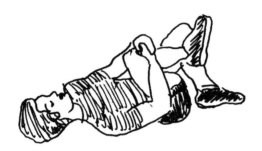

5.   Knee pull

This exercise is done on the back on a firm surface. Both knees are bent with feet resting comfortably on the floor. One leg is taken below the knee and pulled back toward the chest and held between 15-30 seconds. This is done three times and done as needed during the day.

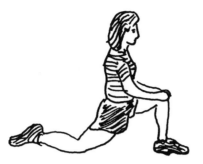

6. Kneeling stretch of the iliopsoas

This exercise is done kneeling on one leg with the other leg pulled back. With the upper body vertical and erect, without bending the head forward, the body is shifted forward stretching the thigh and groin for 15-20 seconds. This is repeated 5-20 times twice a day.

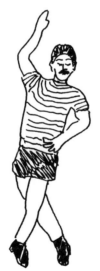

7. Stretching the quadratus lumborum

This exercise is done standing with hands on the hips. One leg is crossed in front of the other rests on the floor. The hips are bent forming a "C" and stretching the other side of the body. This is done three times and repeated as needed during the day.

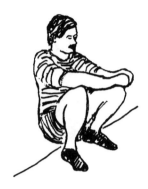

8.   Squat stretch

This stretch opens up the pelvic floor. Squatting on both feet with the back supported against the wall without your 'sit-bones' touching the floor. When there is no discomfort, this pose can be done for 1 + minutes or longer depending on the advice of your physical therapist or physician. This stretch should not be done if there is any pain in the knees.

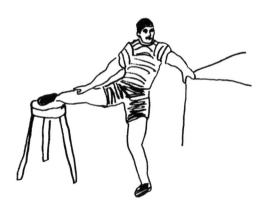

9.   Adductor stretch

In this stretch, the knee that is supporting you is bent slightly in order to increase or decrease the stretch on the inner thigh. The leg that is stretched out is placed on a stool. This should be held for 30 seconds or longer. Change leg after one adductor is stretched to stretch the other adductor. This stretch should not be done if there is any pain experienced in the knees.

Self-treatment of trigger points

When possible we teach patients how to do trigger point release on themselves, usually on the outside of their body, throughout their abdomen and inner thighs. An instrument called a *Theracane* can help in releasing trigger points outside the body. The *Theracane* looks like a funny kind of cane with balls at both ends. One can hold the cane at one end while pushing the ball at the other end of the cane into a trigger point. A tennis ball or foam roll can also be used to assist in some trigger point release.

Sawyer self-administered Myofascial/Trigger Point Release technique

Most patients can do self-administered treatment on the *abdominals* or muscles above the pubic bone, and on the *adductors* or the muscles of the inner thigh. This self-administered treatment, developed by Tim Sawyer our senior physical therapist, can be helpful and should be demonstrated and guided by a physical therapist knowledgeable in this technique.

Patients are instructed to sit in a comfortable chair making it easy to reach their *adductors* and *abdominals*. *Abdominals* can also be reached lying down. Patients are shown how to locate the taut bands of trigger points or tender points on the *abdominals* and *adductors* by systematically feeling these muscles for any tender or painful spots. These tender spots may or may not refer pain into the pelvic floor.

When a tender spot is found, gentle but firm pressure is applied for between 60-90 seconds. When pressure has been applied to all of the tender spots, lotion or oil is applied to the whole length of the inner thigh and to the abdominal area above the pubic bone and these areas are massaged in a gentle but firm sweeping motion. Sometimes the patient is shown how to do skin rolling in which the skin above the inner thigh and above the pubic bone is systematically held in a gentle pinch and rolled or kneaded like kneading dough.

There are some internal trigger points in some patients that can be accessed by the patients themselves. In men, these are usually found in and around the anal sphincter and a little inside of it as well. In women, trigger points that can be worked with at home are found at the opening of the vagina as well as internally close to the opening, and in and around the anal sphincter. The physical therapist doing the myofascial release generally indicates what trigger points the patient can work on at home. Self administered myofascial release should always be done under the supervision of a physical therapist or physician.

Pros and Cons of Our Treatment

We tell new patients who are considering our program about the positive and negative aspects of our treatment.

The cons

Ours is the slow fix, not the quick fix

On the negative side, *ours is the slow fix, not the quick fix.* Our intention is to provide your sore and irritated pelvic muscles and structures with an opportunity to heal. Our method for doing this is 'low tech' and not 'high tech.' During the first 4 months of treatment we ask you to do a good hour of relaxation daily. We tell our patients that our program is like getting a pilot's license you have to put in the hours. Furthermore, you are instructed to practice relaxing the habitual tension in your pelvic floor many times a day by doing *Moment-to-Moment Paradoxical Relaxation*. This is not a small matter.

Myofascial/Trigger Point Release can be painful at first

It is not uncommon during the first several sessions of *Myofascial/ Trigger Point Release* inside the pelvic floor, for there to be flare-ups of symptoms, often between one to three days in length.

Our treatment is inconvenient

Our treatment tends to be inconvenient in that it requires traveling to appointments. The number of actual visits to the doctor or physical therapist who is doing the myofascial release component of treatment varies between approximately ten to thirty visits. Instruction in *Paradoxical Relaxation* averages between six and twenty visits. Home practice, which includes specific stretches and relaxation, must be done daily, and can often take up to an hour. In short, receiving and practicing elements of our protocol is time-consuming and inconvenient.

Insurance often does not cover treatment

Health insurance usually covers some but often does not reimburse all components of our treatments. To date, medical insurance usually covers diagnostic and routine office visits but is spotty in its reimbursement of relaxation training and physical therapy for pelvic pain

Our treatment does not help everybody

While we believe that our treatment is by far the best method to resolve the chronic pelvic pain syndromes in general, our treatment does not help everybody.

The only way to know the effectiveness of treatment is to do it

The full effectiveness of cannot be known until after it is actually done and the effects are evaluated. We always evaluate the appropriateness of our treatment according to a patient's symptoms and recommend it when it is clear that there is no gross pathology and according to our experience, the patient is likely to benefit. In other words even if you fit our criteria as an appropriate candidate, there is no way of determining the level of effectiveness of our treatment for you until you do it earnestly and observe the results.

The pros

Our treatment does not use medication, surgery, or invasive procedures

Our approach does not use of drugs or surgery or invasive procedures. In fact our goal is to help patients off of all drugs. Every patient is examined with a traditional urologic approach and disorders of infection, obstruction, or neurological abnormality are treated appropriately.

No known significant side effects

To our knowledge no one we have seen has suffered any sustained side effect from our treatment. Patients often experience pain, especially at the beginning of the physical therapy part of treatment. This pain, however, tends to diminish as therapy proceeds.

The purpose of our clinics is to make you independent of doctors and health professionals–the majority of treatment is done at home

We teach you how to help yourself. Both in the relaxation training and in many aspects the physical therapy aspect of our protocol, we act as consultants and you are the one responsible to do the treatment.

Whenever possible we enlist the help of a partner. Typically, if a partner is willing, he or she will come in at the beginning sessions of *Myofascial/ Trigger Point Release* and will be instructed in how to administer the trigger point release at home. This helps reduce costs and the inconvenience of having to come to the doctor's or therapist's office so frequently.

When someone has no partner, on a case by case basis, we can prescribe an *internal myofascial wand*, an experimental internal trigger point wand. We have said elsewhere that we do not have FDA approval for this wand and it is used only through prescription at Stanford; where it has been approved for use by the human subjects' committee. This wand requires careful instruction on its use. While we are still evaluating its efficacy, it is possible to use the wand carefully to reach and deactivate internal trigger points that cannot be reached by oneself alone. This wand is a boon to those who live remote from a professional competent in the Stanford Protocol.

Our protocol can help a select group of patients significantly reduce their symptoms or become essentially symptom free

The most important benefit is that our protocol has the real possibility of helping selected individuals with pelvic pain significantly reduce their symptoms or essentially be symptom free. Furthermore as symptoms reduce, a continued improvement in symptoms tends to be ongoing with many patients if they sincerely comply with the protocol and competently manage their response to stress.

CHAPTER 7

FREQUENT CONCERNS

There are certain questions that patients ask about issues including sex, work, relationship, exercise, pain medication, psychotherapy, and alternative treatments. In this chapter we will address these questions. In addition, we share a perspective that we believe is most helpful while you are in the midst of dealing with pelvic pain and dysfunction.

Keeping Your Perspective and Helping Yourself

Pelvic pain is not your enemy

The more severe your symptoms, the more your life tends to revolve around them. As we have reported, dealing with pelvic pain has the same impact on your life as dealing with heart disease or chronic inflammatory bowel disease. Most patients are anxious and depressed and consider their pelvic pain an alien condition that has invaded their lives.

It is one of the intentions of this book to deal with pelvic pain from a number of different perspectives including a larger, existential, or spiritual one. In this section we will discuss the larger view.

Pelvic pain usually does not occur in someone who feels balanced, relaxed, and happy. It tends to be the expression of what is out of balance, fearful, and out of sorts. Viewed this way, you can consider your pelvic pain and dysfunction an intimate advisor about your life. *Pelvic pain is not your enemy. Consider that pelvic pain is part of the main curriculum of your life and not a distraction from it.* Perhaps your curriculum has to do with learning to listen to your own body, to face and manage your anxiety or to express yourself instead of holding things in. Whatever the lessons that are there for you, their resolution, we believe, can positively influence your healing.

You really do have a choice about how you view your condition

A young man with pelvic pain called us from the New York area. He was greatly distressed about his pain and other symptoms. More than anything he wanted his sexual interest to return, an interest that had waned since the onset of his condition.

"Do you think this is an autoimmune disease?" he asked, as he quoted some information he had read on the internet. This young man, like many of our patients, attempted to discover a solution for his problem by reading the literature and the conflicting views and information that he read on the web. This is a subject for which we offer some advice below.

The theories he read about implicating autoimmunity, occult organisms, nerve entrapment, and neurological pathology tended to offer little supporting evidence or effective treatment. They were largely speculative.

The result of his reading made him more anxious and uncertain than before. The more he read that scared him, the more his pain increased. He didn't know what to believe and yet his thinking tended to see his condition from the worst perspective, a fear-producing view that offered nothing to him while making his condition worse.

Once starting our protocol, a number of our patients decided to stop reading about ideas regarding pelvic pain. "All these theories and speculations about my condition scare me," said one patient. "I have decided not to read any more for now and instead focus on the constructive action I am taking by choosing to begin this treatment." In this way they were choosing to take charge of how they looked at their condition.

The pain is not the worst suffering

It is not the pain that is the deepest source of suffering when someone struggles with a chronic pelvic pain syndrome. If we knew for sure that we were going to get better, most pelvic pain and discomfort, while not being something we would choose, would be okay. We would most likely put up with it all without the kind of angst that attends most people who suffer from pelvic pain. It is the *meaning* you give to the symptoms that causes the real suffering.

It is the catastrophic meaning you give to the symptoms and how the impact of this meaning interacts with the pain and tension that is so difficult in dealing with pelvic pain. Consider the following young man who called us in a great state of anxiety about his condition. He was handsome, accomplished, and wealthy and admired by his peers. Women fell in love with him regularly. His friends loved him. He was successful in his profession. He had it all.

For three years he had experienced pain at the tip of his penis along with some post-ejaculatory discomfort and urinary frequency and urgency. The doctors he was fortunate enough to see told him that they could find nothing wrong and there was nothing to worry about. He believed them. He characterized these symptoms to himself as an insignificant annoyance and went on with his life with little concern.

He then happened to go on the internet and started reading the scary stories of those who suffer from pelvic pain that see no light at the end of the tunnel, and scary theories about what some speculate about pelvic pain. His pain became much worse quickly and he spiraled into a dark and deeply upset state. His sleep became disturbed. He withdrew socially. He began to worry about others abandoning him because of his condition. His pain, from being a minor annoyance, sometimes became unbearable. His life became a living hell.

This went on for quite some time. Then he found our book and as quickly as he spiraled into his dark night of the soul, he came out of it. He became clear about what was wrong with him and both his symptoms and his attitude improved dramatically. He came to one of our clinics and his condition further improved. He began having days of no symptoms. Instead of a negative spiral downward, which we describe as the tension-anxiety-pain cycle, he began a positive spiral out of his hole. His view of his condition and its meaning changed. He stopped his catastrophic thinking and saw the possibility of become free of symptoms. The ups and downs of his physical pain and dysfunction were great influenced by his view of what his symptoms meant.

In his classic book, From *Death Camp to Existentialism,* psychiatrist Victor Frankl observed that while he was in a Nazi concentration camp during the Second World War, he discovered the one thing that the Nazis could not take from him was his choice about how to view things. Frankl was clear in his belief that the way he chose to see things helped him survive. Below we will discuss a strategy to deal with the potpourri of theories and remedies, offered to deal with chronic pelvic pain.

A pessimistic view of your condition can literally cause more pain

We have shown that there is scientific evidence demonstrating that your perspective directly affects your pain. Dr. Richard Gevirtz, one of the investigators who discovered that stress increases the level of electrical activity (and pain) in trigger points, put it this way in a telephone call. He said, "Where people have a clear cut model of what is wrong with them and understand that there is something they can do to help themselves, they de-catastrophize what is going on within them." This changed view may physically lower their pain by reducing the effects of sympathetic nervous system arousal inside their trigger points. *The source of their pain is not independent of their thoughts and feelings."*

A school of psychology called cognitive therapy focuses on helping anxious and depressed individuals identify their habitual negative thinking that triggers or aggravates their depressed or anxious states. From the viewpoint of cognitive therapy, when there is a choice, you are going to feel better when you see the glass is half full instead of half empty. A slew of aphorisms illustrate this point.

- *The only difference between a stepping stone and a stumbling block is what you make of it*

- *A glass full to the middle with water can equally be seen as half full or half empty*

- *When being chased out of town, raise a flag and pretend you are leading a parade*

- *When life gives you lemons, make lemonade*

An optimist and a pessimist

A psychologist wanted to study identical twin children, one of whom was considered to be an optimist and the other a pessimist. The pessimistic child was placed in a room full of toys. The optimistic child was placed in a room filled with horse manure. When the psychologist returned after several hours, he found that the pessimistic child had not moved from his chair. Upon inquiring about why the child had not moved to play with the toys, he replied that he was afraid he might break them. When the psychologist entered the room with the optimistic child, he was surprised to see the child covered with manure and digging through it. "What are you doing?" asked the psychologist. Without hesitating, the optimistic child said, "With all this horse manure, there has got to be pony somewhere."

When we have no physical symptoms, we often can tolerate habitual negative ways of thinking. With a condition like a headache in the pelvis that is so intimately tied up with our thinking, our habitual, negative ways of thinking are less benign. They can increase our level of suffering.

Catastrophic thinking only makes you more miserable and is usually not true

Catastrophic thinking is a name given to a pessimistic and negative way of interpreting an event in which you always imagine the worst. The following example of catastrophic thinking illustrates our point. Imagine you feel a little more rectal discomfort than usual when sitting. From this awareness you think that perhaps the doctor has missed a mass in your prostate gland that might be cancerous. You then imagine having surgery in which they have to remove your prostate and you become impotent, incontinent, and that you eventually die despite the removal of the cancer. You imagine that during your dying no one wants to take care of you and you die alone.

This kind of thinking is not uncommon in certain patients that we see. When you tend toward catastrophic thinking, such thinking often feels unremarkable. The catastrophic thinker has rarely considered that there is an alternative to this way of seeing things. When you think catastrophically, you usually are only dimly aware of the contents of your thoughts, and only become fully aware of them and their effects after further examination.

In catastrophic thinking fear always arises. The thought that something serious is wrong with you sets off an alarm in your body that releases emergency substances like adrenaline and cortisol, readying your body for fight or flight. All of a sudden your thinking creates a physical event inside of you.

When you began "catastrophizing" about the rectal pain, as we described above, you unwittingly made up a story in your mind. You jumped from the present moment to four or five steps in the future when you are diagnosed with prostate cancer. Importantly the steps that you simply assume would lead you to a diagnosis of prostate cancer are extremely unlikely.

Catastrophic thinking is rarely true and creates needless suffering. The fear of cancer or some other problem that has remained undiagnosed is common with men we see who have prostatitis. This common process of catastrophizing pelvic pain and dysfunction can spin someone into an anxiety state in which the tension, anxiety, pain cycle makes the pain worse and adds misery to the already existing pain and dysfunction.

Ironically, during the writing of this section of our book, we received a call from someone on the East Coast who was in the kind of anxiety state we have been describing. He described himself as "going crazy" as he read the accounts of sufferers of pelvic pain on the internet who had not been helped and were wretched and desperate. He said his "pain was through the roof." The day after we had an opportunity to discuss our protocol and understanding about the treatment for chronic pelvic pain syndromes, he reported that not only was he feeling relieved emotionally, but also he expressed his puzzlement because he said his pain diminished substantially since our conversation with him. It is not uncommon for patients we have seen to report a reduction in pain simply from the reassurance they feel that perhaps something can be done to help their condition. To one degree or another, many of our patients not only suffer with pelvic pain and dysfunction but a viewpoint that intensifies their symptoms.

The core treatment we use is aimed at rehabilitating the pelvic muscles and the habit of tensing them. However, it is very important to deal with the negative and anxiety producing thinking that is so typical in patients who have chronic pelvic pain syndromes. While not universally true, people with pelvic pain that we treat tend toward catastrophic thinking even prior to the onset of symptoms. Changing this tendency is essential. Below we discuss issues relating to effectively dealing with the kind of negative thinking that aggravates this condition.

Managing catastrophic and anxiety/pain producing thinking: the use of cognitive therapy

How do you stop the kind of thinking which unnecessarily produces anxiety and feeds the cycle of tension, pain, and anxiety? You must first of all see the real connections between your symptoms and your thinking and entertain the idea that it is possible to change catastrophic thinking. What can be called cognitive therapy labels and identifies negative thinking and helps a patient evaluate the credibility of this thinking so that he or she is not a victim of it. For example, in cognitive therapy a patient will say "I can never do anything right" in response to a frustration they are having or an error they have made. The therapist will reflect, "Let's look at the statement 'I can never do anything right' and evaluate the effect of such a thought on one hand, and to critically evaluate whether there is truth in it on the other." A kind of cognitive therapy used with our patients is helpful in the treatment of the anxiety and depression producing thinking that often arises when people have pelvic pain and dysfunction. Below we share some exercises and processes we use with patients.

Negative thought inventory

The negative thought inventory below is an assessment process that you can use to become aware of the effect of your thoughts on your condition. Choose a three-hour period of time when you tend to feel the worst and pay attention to your thoughts. Use a small tape recorder and record any negative thoughts that occur to you on a minute-by-minute basis. After the thought, choose a number from 0 to 10 as to your level of pain. Some examples of the relevant thoughts could include:

- What is wrong with me?
- The pain is worse (maybe it will never get better)
- Am I ever going to get better?
- How can I go on?

- It just does not stop
- What is going to happen to me?
- Here it is again
- I can't understand why it is worse
- Why me?
- Why am I different than so-and-so?
- Will I ever be normal?
- I am never going to get better
- How can I live my life this way?
- No one will love me like this
- Maybe I have cancer
- Maybe I have a sexually transmitted disease and they have not found it yet
- Maybe I have bacteria or fungus they will never find
- If I only had not had sex with so-and-so

Do your best to record your negative thoughts and their effect on your symptoms. This may not be the most enjoyable exercise but we believe it is instructive in helping you see the frequency of certain thoughts and their effect. When you have recorded fifteen minutes of these thoughts, listen to them at the end of a relaxation period. Notice the level of your pelvic symptoms when hearing these thoughts. Record your reactions and insights after this exercise.

Inquiring into negative and catastrophic thoughts with understanding

Our body responds to the conditions in which we find ourselves. Our body responds to our thoughts as if they were real whether they are or not. A person sees a rope, which triggers the thought that the rope is a snake. This person will likely respond with alarm and anxiety as the body instinctually prepares for the danger of a snake. When he sees the rope and releases himself from the idea that it is a snake, his state of alarm stops and his body relaxes because he discovers there is no danger.

Cognitive therapy is not new. It is a general term that refers to the understanding that thinking in large part, creates the reality we live in. The Buddha is reputed to have stated quite elegantly the basic principle of cognitive therapy in *The Dharmapada*, when he said that we create the world we see through our thoughts. If we think we are victims, we ruin our lives. When our view does not see ourselves as victims, our lives transform.

Cognitive therapy is found in the work of Albert Ellis in his *Rational Emotive Therapy*, and in the work of Aaron Beck, former president of the American Psychological Association and others. *A Course in Miracles*, which is an existential textbook that continues to be popular among those involved in spiritual practice, is a powerful form of cognitive therapy. For instance, in one of the beginning lessons in *A Course in Miracles*, the idea is communicated that meaning does not inhere in anything but it is we ourselves who give meaning to everything we see. The year long course offers daily lessons to help students of the Course take back control over what they think.

The best form of cognitive therapy, in our opinion, is offered in the work of Byron Katie who provides an approach to disarming irrational and negative thinking by means of a process that one can do oneself. This is the approach we recommend. Her method, which we have adapted to dealing with the negative thoughts around pelvic pain, offers a way of becoming free from habitual negative and catastrophic thinking.

Step One: Finding the core thought

The key to disarming the catastrophic thinking related to pelvic pain and dysfunction involves first identifying the core thought that your fear and anxiety rests on.

Most physicians rarely have the time or inclinations to delve into the kinds of thinking that are common to people with pelvic pain. Typically, the person with prostatitis or other chronic pelvic pain syndromes lives in a dark world of negative thoughts that is rarely shared with anyone. Each negative thought is taken to be real by the body as it contracts against the scary world created by the thought. These scary thoughts are like gasoline on the fire of the pelvic pain inflaming the pain and the cycle of tension, anxiety and pain.

Formulating the core thought as a statement and not a question

The negative thought inventory is a rich source of the core thoughts fueling much suffering in pelvic pain syndromes. The cognitive therapy process works best with core thoughts that are simple declaratory statements. It is for this reason that we ask patients to write down these thoughts in the form of sentences. Instead of the thought "will I ever be normal," the reformulation of the thought turns out to read, "I will never be normal." Instead of the thought, "will I ever be able to enjoy sex again?" the reformulated sentence is "I will never be able to enjoy sex again."

Formulating the core thought as a definite statement and not simply a possibility

It is also useful to take the catastrophic thoughts that appear tentative and make them definitive. The thought "Maybe I'm going to be in pain for the rest of my life" then becomes "I'm going to be in pain for the rest of my life."

Both making the negative thinking into statements and making them as if they are stating a certainty are framing them in the way in which the body hears them. This reformulation makes these thoughts much easier to deal with when their validity is questioned by the process we use.

Step Two: Face the core thought with openness and curiosity

Like the pain, the negative thoughts are not your enemy. They come from a frightened person's struggle to protect him or herself. The thought of consciously facing one's negative thinking can appear daunting and depressing. Our approach, however, in clearly formulating the core negative thoughts and then examining their validity, usually lightens their impact. In learning to face and evaluate the validity of the negative thinking, we can get control over them.

We tell our patients to face their negative thinking with curiosity and an interest in seeing whether the thoughts are true. Consider your negative thinking as unexamined propositions that may turn out to not be what you think they are. Meet your negative thoughts with openness and understanding.

How to evaluate the validity of the core thoughts from your heart

Experiment with bringing your attention to the feeling in your chest and heart area. Feel the breath and the sensation in your chest as the air comes in and out. With your eyes closed and your attention on your heart and chest area, say your name and feel the feeling in the chest. For example you might say, "My name is John" or "My name is Lindsey" and then you feel the sensation in your chest of truthfully saying your name.

Now keep your attention in your chest area and finish the sentence. "My name is_____" but with a false name. If your name is John, see how it feels in your chest to say that your name is Walter or Dennis. You will probably feel a little tightening or strangeness in your chest. Experiment with feeling your chest as you say your true occupation (i.e., I am an engineer) and then notice the feeling in your chest when you don't tell the truth (i.e., I am a baker or kindergarten teacher).

The point of this exercise is to feel your body's reaction to what is true and what is not true. The body can help you address the validity of your negative thoughts. Refer to the sensation in your body as you address the questions below.

Examining the validity of the core thought

After you have identified the core thought (it is useful to write the thoughts and the answers to the questions down on paper), ask the following questions to yourself about the thought. Feel the area in and around your chest and respond to the questions from this area. In other words, your answers should agree with the feeling in your chest area.

Question your core thought as follows:

1. What is the evidence I have for this core thought?
2. Using this evidence, can I say for sure that this thought is true?
3. What happens physically inside me when I believe that this thought is true?
4. What happens to my self esteem when I believe that this thought is true?
5. What happens to my experience of my life force, my generosity, and love when I believe this thought?
6. What has been the effect of this thought or this kind of thought on my life in the past?
7. What would happen to my life if I simply were incapable of thinking this thought or this kind of thought?
8. What is the opposite kind of thought to this one?

We ask our patients to notice the effect of this questioning on their mood and the impact that this thought has upon them. Catastrophic and negative thinking has usually been practiced for a long time. Doing this questioning process needs to be done often during the day as these kind of thoughts arise very often. It is possible for this process to help reduce the level of anxiety suffering that attends pelvic pain and dysfunction.

Our description of this process is usually not sufficient to become proficient at it. We teach this method in our monthly six day clinics. Information specifically about this cognitive therapy work can be found at www.thework.org and in Byron Katie's excellent book *Loving What Is*, published by Harmony Books in 2002. Listening to the audio version of the book on cassette tape or CD is often more effective than reading the book as one can hear the actual interaction been Katie and people she is working with.

The advanced use of Paradoxical Relaxation: distinguishing between what fearful thoughts arise and the tensions related to such thoughts

Cognitive therapy focuses on the content of what you are thinking. Edmund Jacobson discovered that each negative thought has its own characteristic muscular posture. This means, for example, that when you think the thought "maybe I will never get over this pain," your shoulders rise, your diaphragm pulls in, your jaw tenses and your anal sphincter contracts, your forehead furrows, and your eyes look down. All anxiety-producing thoughts tend to recruit their own characteristic muscle tensions.

While each negative thought tends to have its own characteristic set of muscle tensions, in general, each thought tends to elicit a certain visual mental picture that causes the eyes to tense and to look in a certain direction. For example when you have the thought, "maybe I will never get over this pain," you may repeatedly have a picture of yourself disabled in bed or all alone as an old person. This mental picture is a key to the negative thought and has its own subtle tensions of the small muscles of the eyes.

As someone advances in *Paradoxical Relaxation*, we begin training and identifying these patterns of muscle tension associated with negative thinking. We practice relaxing these tensions along with doing the cognitive therapy described above.

The woman we described earlier who compulsively imagined killing her child learned this procedure of identifying and letting go of muscle tensions associated with this horrific thought. In doing so she freed herself from the guilt and fear that was stimulated by this thought.

It is important to become aware of and to gain control over negative thinking, especially the thinking that is part of a habit of tensing the pelvic muscles. For some individuals, it can be life changing to be able to do this.

What to do about the conflicting (often scary and disheartening) information on the web about your condition

We are often asked about other theories regarding the nature of chronic pelvic pain from people suffering with pelvic pain, a subject we touched upon earlier. Many of these individuals are already in an anxiety state and are looking for some kind of reassurance or guidance as to the nature of their condition and the best course of treatment. When they go on the internet, they read about various theories contending that chronic pelvic pain may be an autoimmune disorder, a condition in which occult bacteria are yet to be discovered, or a deteriorating neurological pelvic condition. These theories do what we have described earlier. They tend to promote fear and helplessness in the sufferer.

When you have pelvic pain, it is deeply disturbing to read theories which promote fear, helplessness, and confusion or hear stories of people who are not doing well with their pain or dysfunction. When you have pain and dysfunction, you usually feel some degree of anxiety and helplessness which is often exacerbated by these kinds of theories. Some of our patients have asked us whether they should ignore the ideas that they read on the web or simply avoid the internet websites devoted to pelvic pain. Others have asked us if there is some way to find out if in fact they have the problem that these theories purport.

If a theory or an idea about your condition carries some course of action or treatment to help you without unacceptable risks, then it may be an idea that merits your careful consideration. You may wish to investigate the efficacy of such a course of treatment along with the risks and costs.

If the theory, on the other hand, carries with it (a) *no course of treatment or action* to be done to help or protect you, or if its treatment carries dangers you are not willing to risk, or (b) it offers some *non-definitive* evidence, and (c) it *only helps to create fear, doubt, and disempowerment* in your life, we suggest you tell yourself, "This is someone's theory. There is no definitive proof for it. It offers nothing to help me or protect me what treatment it offers carries unacceptable risks. It creates fear and doubt in me. It is okay for me to disregard it as somebody's unproven idea which I will consider if there emerges substantial evidence and/or something to do about it. Therefore I can ignore it as simply someone's unproven idea."

This kind of self-talk is the practice of cognitive therapy. Using cognitive therapy about ideas that tend to promote catastrophic thinking is particularly important because, as we have discussed, anxiety tends to increase symptoms.

Faith

Faith is something that is usually discussed in church about matters that are spiritual. It is rarely discussed in a doctor's office as part of a medical condition. When you have faith, you have confidence that somehow everything is okay. When you have faith, even though you don't know how things will turn out, you feel assured that you don't have to know. You trust that things will simply turn out all right.

Faith is a frame that you hold up and through which you look at your life. It is an attitude that you bring to situations whose outcomes are not immediately clear. Faith is a willingness to believe that even though you don't see the light at the end of the tunnel, there is light there. The great poet Rainer Maria Rilke wrote to a young poet who was upset about his lack of facility and success in poetry. Rilke told the young poet to *have patience with what was not resolved within him and to embrace the very questions and unresolved issues themselves without trying to figure out answers.* It was in living in the questions, in being fully present in the midst of difficulties, Rilke wrote him, that he could live his way into the answers.

The 'gift' of pelvic pain and the four Zen horses

While no one would wish pelvic pain on anyone, it can be seen as a gift in that it pushes us beyond what we normally would do to take care of ourselves. It demands that we do whatever it takes to get relief. The following ancient typology of the four Zen horses from the lore of Zen Masters illustrates this point.

The first Zen horse moves as soon as you jump on its back. No whip or word is required. This horse knows what has to be done and takes off as soon as you mount it. *The second Zen horse* takes off when it sees the shadow of your raised whip. While it is not as eager to move as the first horse, it takes only a hint of the whip to get it going. *The third Zen horse* moves when it feels the light sensation of your whip and the pressure of your heels against the sides of its stomach. It is less anxious to move and requires some physical evidence of your intention to make it move. *The fourth Zen horse* will only move when it feels the sting of your whip in the marrow of its bones.

Most of us are the fourth horse. Most of us only buy an umbrella when it is raining and grease a wheel only when it squeaks loudly. Those who come to us with pelvic pain and dysfunction usually do so after these symptoms scare them, or begin to deeply intrude in their lives.

Even when there is pain and dysfunction, most patients are only willing to do our demanding protocol when they are at their wits end. Their motivation comes from feeling that they can't go on in the same way that they have been going. When the pain is intermittent or the impact of the symptoms is minimal, patients tend to be less willing to do what we believe it takes to deal with chronic pelvic pain syndromes. When patients are looking for the "quick fix" we encourage them to see if they can find it elsewhere and return to us if they don't. Patients who have not reached a point of some degree of exasperation tend not to be good candidates for our approach because they are not ready to expend the effort and focus necessary for our protocol to have a chance to help them.

Suffering as grace

Ram Dass was one of the spiritual teachers of young people in the 1960's and has remained as a luminary to many since that time. Over the last few decades, Ram Dass proposed the idea that suffering can be seen as grace or a gift. 'Suffering as grace' means that you acknowledge that even though you wouldn't choose to have the suffering you are dealing with, nevertheless it turns out to be something that may have in it the possibility of transforming your life.

Usually the awareness that suffering can be seen as grace is perceived after the suffering has resolved itself. Nevertheless, many people interested in wisdom traditions and spiritual practices use the idea of suffering as grace as something through which they look at their life difficulties.

Ram Dass also introduced a related idea which we have touched upon that whatever difficulties you may be facing in a particular moment are not distractions from the 'curriculum' of your life, but are the main part of the curriculum itself. Most people believe that their condition has taken their attention away from what they really want to be doing. When you look at your difficulties as your main curriculum you bring an entirely different attitude to them. This has the power to transform your difficulties because you stop resisting or hating them.

What does this mean for you if you are suffering from pelvic pain? We think that it is useful to view your condition as one of the 'main courses' that you are enrolled in, in the 'university' called your life. We are not suggesting that you have deliberately brought this pain into your life that you want it there, or you shouldn't resolve it as soon as possible. We are suggesting the idea that if you do have pelvic pain and dysfunction, that you acknowledge that you have it and ask yourself the questions. What is it asking from me? What lesson does my current predicament contain for me? Am I listening?

Taking a long view: managing your expectations

Unrealistic expectations will make you anxious and increase your pain and suffering. In our view, pelvic pain and dysfunction does not come about out of the blue, even though in some cases it may seem so. In our experience, even with our most successful patients, symptoms take a significant amount of time to resolve.

We suggest that patients who begin our protocol give themselves a good year in which to do our protocol before expecting symptoms to become reliably better. While not everyone benefits from our treatment, the majority who do, experience a substantial improvement or an abatement of symptoms. It may require a considerable period of time for this to happen.

Taking a year does not mean that patients will not experience a benefit quite soon after beginning treatment. Giving yourself a year means understanding that typically a person's condition normally fluctuates, especially at the beginning of treatment.

We suggest to patients not to celebrate when they are feeling better, or despair when they are feeling worse. Typically during the course of treatment, patients can have twenty or thirty flare-ups, each followed by an improvement of symptoms. Symptom intensity can go up and down often because it is as if we are renovating a building while still living in it.

We have touched on the conflict between resting the pelvic muscles and having the need to use them to function in life. In an ideal world we would send the pelvic muscles to a tropical island for a long rest. Unfortunately this is not possible. We cannot avoid the stresses and strains that interfere with our healing and trigger symptoms. We tell our patients to give their pelvic floor lots of room to go through its gyrations as they do physical therapy, and the two forms of *Paradoxical Relaxation*.

Learning to be unconditional with yourself

One of the major lessons for those dealing with pelvic pain and dysfunction is learning to be unconditional with yourself and do what ever it takes to help yourself. By unconditional, we are referring to an attitude of "I am going to be present with myself while I have this problem. I will be here for myself without limitations or conditions and do whatever it takes, for as long as it takes, to help myself."

Most of us have never completely devoted ourselves to our own care. *The protocol that we use requires time and patience.* We will often tell patients that while we have some general parameters of how long it takes for the symptoms to abate, when the protocol works, it will take as long as it takes. People who come to our treatment with this attitude of unconditionality seem to do the best.

Learning to be a witness to yourself

When you have pelvic pain, it can become the major focus in your life. Earlier, we described how we teach our patients in the relaxation training how to be a witness to the experience of tension and discomfort as a way of reducing it and letting it go. Daniel Goleman in his book, *Emotional Intelligence*, describes being able to be a witness of yourself as a master aptitude in dealing with your own emotions and those of others. When you can be a witness to yourself, you can step outside and objectively see yourself.

The *Paradoxical Relaxation* taught in our protocol requires that you feel and allow the experiences in your pelvic muscles without interfering with them in any way. *Being a witness to your pain and discomfort is usually necessary to relax it.*

The opposite of being a witness to your pain or discomfort is getting lost in it. Goleman refers to being lost in your emotions, rather than witnessing them as 'emotional high-jacking.' When you are emotionally high-jacked your emotions sit in the driver's seat of your life and take you on the ride of their choosing. When you are 'emotionally high-jacked' by your anger, you can punch someone in the face or do or say something that your rational ethical self would never do. When you are angry and not high-jacked by your anger, but witnessing it, you feel the anger and contain it and don't 'come from it'. Your anger does not decide what you do. You do.

In the same way when you are high-jacked by your discomfort and the fear that often attends a headache in the pelvis, your pain, and fear sit in the driver's seat of your life. You get lost in the catastrophic thinking that is associated with such high-jacking. As a reflex, you tense up against the pain even more which causes more pain. You make a difficult situation even worse.

When people are in pain, they tend to forget that they were ever out of pain. And when people are out of pain, they can hardly remember being in pain. We have seen repeatedly that a patient can be out of pain for months. Then circumstances conspire to push them above the symptom threshold and they are back in the old familiar territory of pelvic pain and dysfunction. The tension-anxiety-pain cycle reasserts itself and they lose perspective. They stop witnessing what is happening.

When symptoms go away, most patients find it hard to remember the intensity of their emotions when they were symptomatic. Instead of catastrophic thoughts, they have "anastrophic" thoughts—thoughts that say "my suffering is over forever—it is gone away, never to return."

In both the tendency toward catastrophic thinking when flare-ups occur, or anastrophic thinking when symptoms abate, perspective is lost. The ability to witness is lost. The catastrophic thinking that can occur with a flare-up involves suffering. Equally, the anastrophic thinking that the pain is gone forever is setting up acute suffering and disappointment when there is a flare-up. Both are unrealistic. Both need to be witnessed and worked with so that you save yourself unnecessary suffering while in treatment.

The patients we have seen who have agreed to and later suffered from heroic measures like pelvic surgeries, for the most part, were seized by their emotions. In agreeing to these kinds of interventions, they were often in a state of near panic and desperation. "Just do something—anything to make my symptoms stop" is the message they brought to the doctor. Unfortunately, they often found a doctor willing to participate in their desperate need to do something by experimenting with interventions and surgeries that often left them worse off.

When you are willing to be a witness to your pain and anxiety you are expressing your faith that somehow it is all right that in the moment, fear and pain exist in you. In our experience, in that moment of allowing them to simply be there, they tend to relax. Not that we are saying that they all go away. Witnessing tension, anxiety, and pain, however, almost always reduces suffering. As we have examined in the section on *Paradoxical Relaxation*, relaxation occurs with an attitude of 'it is okay for this pain/discomfort/tension to be here as it is.'

Jean Klein, a physician and meditation teacher, noted that the moment that you observe that you are inside a cage, you have stepped out of it. Being the witness to yourself allows you to face fear instead of simply reacting to it by fighting or fleeing. When Walter Cannon observed that the reflex response to danger is fight, flight or freeze, he was commenting on the reflex reaction of the human mammal. When we are willing to witness our unhelpful fight, flight or freeze reaction, we go beyond our automatic animal programming into a higher domain. Here there is a greater possibility of resolving our concern.

How to gauge your progress once you are in treatment

Witnessing and understanding flare-ups help reduce their impact. When our treatment works, within a relatively short time there is usually a decrease in the intensity and frequency of the symptoms interspersed with regular flare-ups. Typically a patient will notice an easing in the discomfort of the pelvic floor during or after the relaxation but the pain or discomfort almost always returns sooner rather than later. The 'windows' of being pain free tend to increase, but the course of healing often is 3 steps forward and 2 steps backward.

If you are in treatment, don't evaluate your progress in *all-or-nothing* terms. Often patients will feel better for short periods and then return back to the old sense of discomfort and dysfunction. When our treatment works, these windows usually increase, lessening the suffering of constant and unremitting pain. As the therapy continues, and as the person learns to relax more deeply, the periods of being pain-free and dysfunction-free increase. Notice if there is a decrease in the *overall* intensity or the frequency of the symptoms. This is a much kinder and at the same time more realistic way of evaluating how your personal healing is going.

Psychotherapy can sometimes make dealing with your condition a little easier

It is our experience that psychotherapy alone does not significantly reduce or eliminate the symptoms of chronic pelvic pain syndromes. That said, there is a use for psychotherapy in an adjunctive and supportive role in dealing with chronic pelvic pain syndromes.

Anxiety about the future which plagues people who have pelvic pain tends to fester when it is suppressed and not given a safe place in which to be expressed. When it is painful to sit, to urinate, or to have sex, many thoughts are stimulated about what this all means and what is going to happen in the future. Unexpressed, this kind of thinking tends to cycle around and around in the kinds of catastrophic thinking we described earlier.

It is often hard for most of us to find friends who can hear our fears and anxieties with any degree of understanding and without reactivity. Many people feel baffled, helpless, and afraid to hear of such strange doings and feelings as go on with people who are suffering with pelvic pain. This is one of the important reasons why people with this condition feel isolated and alone. They feel that they have no one to talk to. They are afraid that if they share their real thoughts and feelings with anyone, no matter how close and caring, that the person won't know what to do with such sharing. In large part they are right.

A safe place to regularly share the burden you carry

Psychotherapy can serve the purpose of having a place to express difficult thoughts and feelings. One of the benefits of psychotherapy is that you are paying someone to be present to hear what is going on someone who has no history with you. The psychotherapist, whom you might see, however, should have both familiarity with and an understanding of your condition and support you in what you are doing about it. Also, the psychotherapist needs to be free from reactivity or fear when hearing what is going on with you.

This kind of psychotherapy can lighten your load a little. When choosing a psychotherapist it is a good idea to find someone who is experienced and who comes recommended. We suggest that patients educate the psychotherapist about their condition by giving them this section of the book to read. It is sometimes advisable for the psychotherapist to consult with someone on our team to learn more about our protocol and the best way the psychotherapist can support it. If you are doing our protocol or are contemplating doing it, it is in your interest to make sure everyone you are working with is going in the same direction. In our view, it is not a good idea to be doing simultaneous treatments that are uncoordinated or in any way, at odds with each other.

We recommend that patients tell the therapist that they want a place to share their feelings and are not looking for advice about what to do about their condition. Psychotherapists are people. They are as likely as anyone else to deal with their own inner discomfort or sense of helplessness upon hearing someone's troublesome situation by trying to 'fix' the problem. This can come in the form of giving advice or making global psychological interpretations about the meaning of the symptoms.

EMDR

Beyond using cognitive and supportive psychotherapy, there is a role in psychotherapy for more specific purposes. Approaches that can be of assistance in the resolution of pelvic pain include Eye Movement Desensitization and Reprocessing (EMDR) for sexual and physical trauma, cathartic therapies in dealing with suppressed emotions, and relationship therapy in working with the interpersonal difficulties that can occur with loved ones.

A small but not insignificant number of patients have tightened their pelvic muscles chronically as a reaction to physical or sexual abuse. Often the tightening up of the pelvic muscles for these patients was part of their way of defending themselves against the trauma reoccurring. "If I open myself up and relax, I will be inviting something bad to happen so I have to remain contracted" or "If I open myself up I will be overwhelmed by the pain inside me" represent the kind of unconscious thinking of some people who have experienced trauma.

We generally refer patients who have had sexual or physical abuse that may be contributing to their pelvic pain to a psychotherapist experienced in EMDR. This method aims to resolve the frozen feelings and memories that occur in a person's life when such feelings and memories were impossible for the person to process at the time the abuse occurred.

Dr. Francine Shapiro discovered that earlier traumatic events seem to loosen their hold on traumatized people when, in a therapeutic environment and guided by a trained therapist, they move their eyes (or attention) rhythmically while talking about the event. EMDR makes use of the fact that parts of the body connected with processing of experience tend to freeze up during a traumatic event and at subsequent times when the event is recalled.

To understand this, recall what you do when you have had a difficult encounter during the day. Typically you will want to talk about it and share it with someone close to you. You do this as a way of 'processing' the difficult experience in order to be able to let it go so that you can be free in the moment again. Imagine what would happen if you had a fight with your boss, your spouse or your friend that was not resolved and you were not able to talk about it with anyone. The experience would feel like something stuck inside you that needs to come out but does not. Being unable to share your thoughts and feelings would most likely feel extremely physically and emotionally uncomfortable.

When someone has been the victim of incest, sexual trauma, or physical assault, the level of distress they feel is multiplied by many orders of magnitude in comparison to a simple interpersonal upset. Consciousness tends to freeze during this kind of event as if to control or contain it. From the viewpoint of the traumatized person the trauma is perceived to be too big to handle. In order to protect itself from being overwhelmed, the body/mind tends to freeze up around the trauma.

EMDR helps unfreeze a person's frozen consciousness around a traumatic event. The methodology of EMDR allows the event to be processed in the same way you would process an upset with your boss by talking to a friend. The processing that occurs in EMDR around traumas such as sexual and physical abuse, however, tends to be much more dramatic than your discussion with your friend about the upset with your boss. Tears, shuddering, grief, and anger can arise in the EMDR processing. Such reactions were suppressed during the traumatic event. As the event continues to be recalled while the eyes, ears or senses focus on movement, the trauma can be processed and resolved.

The usefulness of cathartic psychotherapy

Any difficult life situation that does not allow a person to express strong emotions or feelings can result in a person chronically tightening the muscles of the pelvic floor. For instance we have seen patients whose triggering event appears to be the suppression of feelings around the death of a loved one or some other life-shaking loss. We speculate that the pelvic floor muscles are tightened because the emotions are not being expressed.

Catharsis-oriented psychotherapies can be of use in helping our troubled patients vent suppressed emotions. In this way a major obstacle to treatment can be removed.

Reichian therapy, Bioenergetics, and Holotropic Breath Work

There are several psychotherapeutic methods that are useful in allowing suppressed emotions to be expressed. Reichian therapy, bioenergetics, rebirthing and holotropic breath work are all methods that have grown up on the periphery of standard "talking" psychotherapy. They are methods that aim specifically at providing an environment and methodology that can assist a person in directly expressing emotions that have been suppressed.

Wilhelm Reich M.D., the inventor of Reichian therapy, was particularly interested in what he called the muscular "armoring" of the pelvis and the effect of stopping the energy and feeling from moving through it. Reich developed a powerful psychotherapy able to unlock suppressed emotions.

Alexander Lowen, M.D., a New York psychiatrist popularized *Reichian therapy* in a form called *bioenergetics*. Lowen wrote several popular books from the 1950's through the 1990's. Bioenergetics is also very effective in dealing with suppressed emotions.

Stanislaus Grof, M.D., developed *Holotropic Breath Work* as a way of reconstituting the therapeutic aspects of the psychedelic experience without the use of drugs. Grof was a researcher who studied the effects of psychedelic substances and was deeply moved by the power of these drugs to produce positive therapeutic effects. *Holotropic Breath Work* is often done in groups, lasts a number of hours per session, and encourages patients to let down and allow their deepest feelings to arise and be expressed. This too is a powerful methodology.

A full presentation of the theoretical underpinnings and methods of Reichian therapy, bioenergetics, and Holotropic Breath Work is beyond the scope of this book. We believe these modalities can be useful in helping to resolve emotional difficulties that some of our patients may have that interfere with their relaxation of the pelvic muscles.

Sexual shame and guilt

The issues of shame and guilt with regard to sex sometimes may be related to pelvic pain and are appropriate subjects to be dealt with in psychotherapy that is adjunctive to our protocol. Numerous studies have demonstrated that there is a higher incidence of pelvic pain among women who have been sexually traumatized. While studies have not focused so much on men, in our experience, issues around sex are often related to the onset of pelvic pain. Let's explore briefly the likely relationships between sexual anxiety, shame, guilt, and pelvic pain.

The pursuit of sexual pleasure, the frustration humans often experience in achieving it, the turmoil that often attends it in interpersonal relationships, and the religious injunctions against it, are all issues that loom large in human life.

It is our speculation that on a psychological level, tension in the pelvic muscles can be an example of a defense, expressed physically, that is related to sex. Here are some examples. We saw a forty year old woman, who was raped by her father when she was fifteen. She vowed "never to allow anything to come into her vagina again." Twenty five years later she came to see us suffering with vaginal pain. Our treatment included teaching her to relax her pelvis. Her traumatic history, however, fought against the goal of our treatment. Without resolving the psychological issues that continued to support her chronic pelvic tension, her situation, and treatment would be like pressing on the gas pedal with one foot and the brake with the other.

There was 18 year-old man who was nervous about sex. He had never masturbated or had any sexual activity in his life. He began having intense sexual dreams, which frightened him, and he tightened up his pelvic muscles as a way of trying to control the sensations and emotions that were arising. After several months, he went to his family doctor and reported having urinary frequency and urgency and pain above the pubic bone. Asking this young man to relax his pelvic muscles without helping him resolve his sexual anxiety would not be a viable therapeutic strategy.

We have also seen a number of men and women who had been involved in extramarital affairs and later reported the onset of pelvic pain after them. After seeing a physician to rule out sexually transmitted diseases, they came to see us. In our meetings with them it emerged they suffered from shame and fear about their extramarital experience. It has been our speculation that they focused tension in their pelvic muscles in some unconscious way of protecting themselves in response to this shame and fear.

In these and other examples, the sexual thoughts and experiences of some patients have been strongly associated with the onset of their symptoms. These examples represent a small percentage of our patients. Nevertheless, for certain patients these issues are crucial, and resolving them makes it possible for symptoms to abate.

Pleasure anxiety and when feeling safe feels scary

Psychotherapy is useful in addressing what can be called "pleasure anxiety." Pleasure anxiety refers to an aversion toward pleasure because it triggers an unconscious fear that something bad might happen. Pleasure anxiety is often seen in individuals who have suffered some life-changing trauma like the death of a parent.

Here is an example to explain pleasure anxiety. A patient with pelvic pain experienced the suicide of her mother at a time in her life when our patient was happy and carefree. The news of her mother's death occurred suddenly and shocked her. From the time of her mother's death she remained nervous and wary. In her mind, the experience of being happy and carefree was somehow connected to a terrible event happening.

It was for this reason that she complained that she could never relax. With a psychotherapist, while in therapy, she had noticed that as she grew older and explored her life she seemed to be uncomfortable 'feeling good.' She reported that invariably when she felt a sense of contentment, negative thoughts about things that might happen in the future would come to her mind and her good mood evaporated. Moreover, she reported that she felt strangely naked when her pelvic pain would subside. Her treatment involved a focus on tolerating pleasure and accepting the absence of anxiety.

The core of our treatment for pelvic pain is training our patients to profoundly relax their pelvic muscles. *You can't relax the pelvic muscles without relaxing everywhere else in the body. Paradoxical Relaxation means that you 'un-defend yourself.' It means that you allow yourself to be at ease, to feel good, and to let go of vigilance.*

Our treatment bumps up against psychological patterns that refuse to let go of psychological defenses. When patients are at a plateau in which their symptoms stop improving it is often helpful to facilitate a dialogue between the part of the patient who wants to improve and the part that seems unable to move ahead. What often emerges from these dialogues is the fear of the unknown that is imagined if there is no more pain or dysfunction.

Sex and prostatitis

In general, most cases of prostatitis affect a man's experience of sex to one degree or another. In bacterial prostatitis the pain and urinary dysfunction usually have an effect on sexual functioning or pleasure.

After this acute episode is over, the bacteria are eliminated from the prostate and the infection is resolved. There is commonly no further impact upon sex. In chronic bacterial prostatitis, we have seen sexuality being affected during acute episodes like those in simple bacterial prostatitis. This impact tends to go away when the infection/ inflammation is cured as it does with bacterial prostatitis. In other words, in both bacterial and chronic bacterial prostatitis, sexuality tends to be impacted while a man is symptomatic and sexuality is not affected once the symptoms clear up.

In nonbacterial prostatitis/CPPS, which represents approximately 95% of all of the cases, sexual functioning and pleasure is usually affected. If the symptoms in chronic pelvic pain syndrome are intermittent, generally speaking sexuality is only affected when other symptoms are present.

When symptoms are experienced chronically, men usually have pain or discomfort during or after ejaculation. Typically, a man with CPPS experiences increased aching, discomfort, or pain after intercourse lasting from a few hours to a few days. This experience takes its toll, and while most men continue to experience sexual desire, it is dampened by the sense that there will be pain or discomfort afterward.

It is not uncommon for some men to complain of a reduction in sexual interest, problems performing sexually, or a diminution in the strength of their erections. We do not believe that there is a physical basis for these complaints. Rather it is our view that the man's attitude and emotions and/or anticipation of pain can have a powerful effect on the reduction of sexual interest and pleasure. Furthermore, the responses of the spinal cord reflexes are dampened by pelvic discomfort.

Counter to traditional advice it is sometimes useful to reduce the frequency of sexual activity

The same traditional idea that prescribes antibiotics for prostatitis often includes the recommendation to increase frequency of ejaculation. We have seen many men who have been told by their urologists to increase the frequency of ejaculation to relieve "congestions" of the prostate gland and the seminal vesicles. This is largely folklore as there is no evidence that pelvic pain comes about because of any such congestion. Nevertheless, many men are given this advice or hear of it and follow it. Patients often ask advice about sexual activity because of their concern about their discomfort during or after ejaculation. In addition, flare-ups are common after increasing the number of times they ejaculate. Not only is increased frequency of ejaculation not indicated, but also in our view it often exacerbates the problem.

Orgasm as a pleasure spasm

The reason that there is often an increase in discomfort during or after sexual activity in men with chronic pelvic pain syndromes is as follows. Ejaculation causes strong contractions of the prostate and pelvic muscles about once a second. *Orgasm is a pleasure spasm.* There is a significant increase in nervous system arousal during sexual activity. The pleasure spasm of orgasm in the form of the increased series of contractions during orgasm will tighten the pelvic muscles further. This increased tightening temporarily adds tension to an already tense area which doesn't relax well and it tends to throw the patient further above the symptom threshold. After a while, the muscles relax and return to their baseline level, the normal state of the pelvic floor reasserts itself (which is back to some degree of pain or discomfort when a man has chronic pelvic pain syndrome). For this reason we do not recommend increasing sexual activity when a man has a pronounced increase in symptoms after sex.

Sometimes it is helpful to do *Myofascial/Trigger Point Release* after sex. Some men have reported that they themselves or their partners gently stretch their pelvic floor muscles after sex, and in combination with relaxation, their post ejaculatory symptoms reduce. Sometimes it is useful to do skin rolling, self massage or insertion of a gloved and lubricated finger in the anus and gently stretch the tightened tissue after sex. It is often useful to do relaxation before sex or relaxation and a hot bath after sex. Some men have escaped the flare up of sexual activity by taking 5 milligrams Valium® before or immediately after sex. The point of all of these strategies is to quiet down the tightening of the muscles after sexual activity. These strategies become less important as the pelvis returns to a more overall relaxed state.

Sometimes it is useful to reduce frequency of ejaculation

Contrary to the common advice some urologists give patients to increase the frequency of ejaculation, we think it more prudent to suggest to patients that they consider reducing the number of times they ejaculate. This is particularly important advice for men who compulsively masturbate. While the experience of ejaculation usually reduces their anxiety and discomfort for a brief while, it often creates more pain or discomfort. When our treatment is effective, as symptoms quiet down, the frequency of sexual activity can return to normal.

Increasing sensuality in the midst of the pain and dysfunction of pelvic pain syndromes

Men in our culture tend to be uncomfortable in acknowledging either to themselves or others their needs for closeness, connectedness, and non-sexual intimacy. In our culture men often hit each other on the back, punch each other on the shoulder, or call each other names. These are ways men express their affection and connection with each other while maintaining the appearance of appropriate manliness.

Many men get their need for love, affection, closeness, and reassurance through sexual intercourse. Not uncommonly, anxious men who are not in a sexual relationship will frequently masturbate as a way of lowering their anxiety. *In a word, sex is often used by men to address needs that are not sexual.*

When men have some form of chronic pelvic pain syndrome, *there are many burdens that they must bear that are not discussed.* Men we see in our clinic frequently complain of their reduced interest in sex. *What is rarely expressed is the fact that when a man has pelvic pain and dysfunction, often discomfort related to sexual activity throws a pall on one of the only ways he can be intimate or relax.*

When the cost of sex is particularly difficult or onerous, we recommend to our patients to choose to cuddle with their partner without the aim of being sexual and having orgasm. We will recommend, for instance, that a man exchange non-sexual massages with his wife, or agree to lie on a couch with his partner and exchange a foot massage. These intimate yet non-sexual moments serve to address the often increased anxiety in a man and helps quiet down the often difficult times that are occurring in the marital relationship.

It is okay to be less sexual for a while

Not uncommonly, some of the men with prostatitis have an idea that their masculinity depends on their ability to have intercourse and satisfy their partner. When we suggest that perhaps they have sex less frequently, these patients may express discomfort and worry at how their partner will react.

We will sometimes suggest that our patient be clear with his partner that he can give her sexual pleasure but will refrain from having orgasm himself. This pleasure might be in the form of sexual massage, or bringing his wife to orgasm without having intercourse. In this way the needs of his relationship, which are often a big concern to our patients, can be met while minimizing a flare-up of symptoms.

None of these measures is ideal

We do not want to give the impression that simply cuddling, or pleasuring one's partner, resolves the sexual issues brought about by prostatitis. These measures are attempts to ameliorate the situation under circumstances that are at best difficult. We understand that the best solution we can offer to the issue of sex and the problems that arise between a man with chronic pelvic pain syndrome and his partner is for his symptoms to get better or go away.

Practice in relaxing the pelvic muscles during sex

We have found that entering into and completing sexual activity while the pelvic muscles are relaxed can help reduce discomfort related to sexual activity. Below we will outline some steps you can take in changing the often unconscious habit of tensing the pelvic muscles before and during orgasm.

Become aware of what goes on in your pelvic muscles during sexual activity:

- Notice if you are anxious in anticipating being sexual.

- Notice if there are any anxieties that occur during sexual activity.

- Notice if there is any sense of urgency in moving toward orgasm or if there is a sense of leisure about it.

- Notice if there is any unnecessary tightening of your pelvic muscles as sexual sensation builds up, as you get close to orgasm or during orgasm.

- Do your best to notice if you add unnecessary tension to the experience of orgasm.

- Notice what happens when you practice the intention of voluntarily reducing your tension during sexual activity.

- Notice if there is any difference in the quality of the orgasm or in your level of discomfort after orgasm by slowing down and relaxing during sexual activity.

Notice without trying to influence what is going on

This practice of noticing what you are actually doing with your pelvic muscles during sex needs to be done *without interfering with it*. First, observe. Then consider the following:

The instructions of *Paradoxical Relaxation* can also be used for changing the habit of squeezing the pelvic muscles during sex. *Your practice of Paradoxical Relaxation will be most clearly seen in your ability to accept and relax with the incompleteness of the sexual experience midway through it.* Men commonly are captured by the impulse to get to the orgasm. This impulse is usually accompanied by pelvic tension and lack of ease. Our recommendation is: *instead of tightening your pelvic muscles and rushing toward orgasm in the way that you might normally be accustomed to do, slow down and feel the subtlety of the sensations along the way.* Doing this is not easy at first and requires a certain discipline and willingness to postpone immediate gratification. We will address below the subject of not making sex an emergency.

Not making sex an emergency

When a man has a high level of tension in his pelvic muscles it is common that he tightens up during sex. Anxiety about performance and "rushing" to the climax is not unusual. When a man squeezes his pelvic muscles at a time when the pelvic muscles naturally contract, there is often a reduction in sexual sensation and an increased likelihood of increased pelvic pain or discomfort afterward.

It is for this reason that we offer the idea of not making sex an emergency. What this means in practical terms is that a man practices the relaxation method of our protocol throughout his sexual experience. This means that he stays in touch with his often unconscious tendency to tighten his muscles during sex and instead of reflexively tightening, he relaxes. *Relaxing during sexual activity means that you allow the genital experience to come to you rather than you try to control it.* This practice of relaxing during sex is unknown territory to most men. Doing this requires being receptive more than being active. It means that anxiety is not in the driver's seat during the sexual act. Relaxing during sex tends to be accompanied by an increased level of physical and emotional sensitivity.

Being in a sexual embrace, while being profoundly relaxed is not a new idea. This attitude has been around for thousands of years and exists today in the practice of what is called 'tantric yoga.' As we will describe in our discussion of managing sexual difficulties with vulvar pain, while tantric yoga has spiritual goals, our purpose in discussing this practice is to help restore the health of the pelvic muscles.

It is important that sex is not an emergency situation. Having sex in a very relaxed way in conjunction with the rehabilitation and relaxation of the pelvic muscles, helps keep the pelvic muscles from going into the heightened level of tension that we believe is responsible for the increased discomfort after intercourse. To repeat, deeply relaxing and being receptive during sexual activity is not easily learned. The impulse is often to do it quickly. Learning to deeply relax while being sexual takes time, patience, and perseverance. Aside from reducing symptoms, this practice has other rewards of increased presence, interpersonal connectedness, and pleasure.

The impact of interstitial cystitis on sex

The bladder is primarily affected in interstitial cystitis (IC) and there is little evidence of any direct 'physical' impairment of sexual functioning in this condition. Unlike vulvar pain, women with IC do not usually report pain upon penetration during intercourse. It is not uncommon, however, for women to have pain during the thrusting phase of intercourse. This makes sense because we often find trigger points in the muscles in and around the bladder and the pelvic floor in women with this condition.

A large impact upon sexuality in patients who have IC undoubtedly relates to the dampening effect of pelvic pain and urinary dysfunction on sexual desire and functioning. That is to say that the consuming intrusion of urinary frequency and urgency, and sometimes chronic pain in the bladder and pelvic floor takes its toll on a person's interest in sex as it takes a toll on a general interest in life. Sexual interest and functioning improve as pain and symptoms abate.

The best prescription in dealing with the negative impact of this condition on sexuality is not different from that of chronic pelvic pain syndrome. The profound relaxation of the pelvic floor, the physical loosening of the muscles and deactivation of the trigger points in the pelvic floor, proper management of diet, and anything else that will quiet down bladder pain, can also simultaneously help sexual pleasure and interest.

As we will discuss in relation to vulvar pain, non-penetrative sexual practices can help in dealing with the negative impact of IC on sexuality. This, in conjunction with physical but non-sexual intimacy including cuddling and massage can be helpful.

Vulvar pain and sexuality

Of all of the varieties of pelvic pain syndromes, vulvar pain tends to have the strongest impact upon a woman's sexual life. The initial complaint of most women with vulvar pain relates to pain associated with intercourse. This problem is most vexing and troublesome because it affects young women who for the most part desire to be in a relationship and have a family. Their vulvar pain impacts either finding a relationship or living happily in one.

The four stages of dyspareunia (pain during intercourse)

It is useful to chart a woman's progress in treatment by the extent to which her sexual activity is affected by her condition. In doing this, it is useful to identify four degrees of dyspareunia (pain during intercourse). Women with vulvar pain, depending on their degree of the pain, report experiencing themselves somewhere in the following stages:

- *Stage one:* A woman can tolerate penetration, thrusting, and the completion of intercourse. However, she experiences some degree of tolerable pain, usually at the beginning of intercourse when her partner enters her vagina.

- *Stage two:* A woman can tolerate penetration, thrusting, and the completion of intercourse with pain throughout.

- *Stage three:* A woman can tolerate penetration but has difficulty tolerating any thrusting. As a rule she cannot complete intercourse. This stage finds a woman generally being avoidant of sex because of the pain.

- *Stage four:* A woman cannot tolerate penetration. A woman who has stage four dyspareunia has simply stopped having intercourse.

Dr. Howard Glazer, associate professor of psychology in obstetrics and gynecology at Cornell Medical College, strongly recommends that women renew non-penetrative sexual practices that lead to orgasm. He encourages couples to engage in sexual activity that does not bring about pain, and yet allows for emotional and sexual intimacy leading to orgasm. This includes clitoral stimulation, mutual masturbation, the use of dildos and vibrators which usually do not irritate the vulva.

Many women with vulvar pain have simply stopped being sexual because of the painful consequences of sexual intercourse. Glazer's advice is aimed at helping a woman 're-sexualize' herself. When women complain that they don't feel interested in sex, Glazer recommends the resumption of non-painful sexual activity aimed at rehabilitating the pelvic muscles and vulvar tissue that have become used to inactivity. Furthermore, Glazer addresses what would be considered the psychological aspect that might be present in the avoidance of sexual activity. This includes dealing with unresolved interpersonal problems that may exist in a relationship that would incline a woman to pull away sexually from her partner and from sex in general. Glazer addresses issues of shame, sexual abuse, self-esteem and self-image, and other psychological factors that might impact on a woman's sexual activity and interest. In this re-sexualizing aspect of Glazer's work, he recommends a book called *Let Me Count the Ways: Discovering Great Sex without Intercourse* by Kline and Robins.

Glazer calls the work he does with the psychological and interpersonal factors involved in vulvar pain "psycho-education," rather than psychotherapy. He is clear that this focus on the psychological is some small part of the picture of vulvar pain but by no means the whole picture. He says that while the psychological and interpersonal factors are a small part of the picture, they loom large enough in some women to determine whether a woman resumes an active and enjoyable sex life.

The 're-sexualization' prescription is not only meant for the psychological and interpersonal health of the woman. Glazer has taken into consideration the fact that there is evidence of a reduction of blood flow into the vulvar area of most women who have vulvar pain. Sexual activity necessarily involves blood flow into the vulva and other parts of the vagina. Glazer's intention in recommending increased non-penetrative and non-irritating sexual activity is to promote vulvar health and prevent the atrophy of blood vessels and other tissue that can be involved in abstinence from regular sexual activity.

We generally advise women with vulvar pain to explore ways of being sexual that will not throw them into a flare-up, yet can allow them some degree of sexual intimacy even when they are symptomatic. We don't pretend that these measures are an answer to the problem. They simply offer the possibility of having some semblance of sexual intimacy while the patient is proactively dealing with her condition.

Women with vulvar pain generally hurt upon their partner's entrance into the vagina. The discomfort also occurs during the thrusting phase of intercourse. With some women, the pain is immediate. With other women, the pain or discomfort comes after sex.

When there is improvement in the condition of a woman with vulvar pain, we suggest that patients experiment with the practice of '*tantra.*' Generally speaking, we suggest this to women who are in the first stage of dyspareunia. *Tantra* allows for a couple to have sexual intercourse with a minimum of movement and irritation to a woman's vulva. This ancient practice prescribes that a man slowly enters inside a woman and once inside that he moves very little. His attention is focused on the sexual sensations in his genitals and in the sexual and sensual connection with his partner. His focus is on relaxing with the combination of sexual pleasure and the sense of incompleteness of holding back from moving toward orgasm.

When the man begins to lose his erection, he will move around to stimulate himself until his erection becomes firmer. He then continues relaxing, directing his attention to the connection between himself and his partner. He remains receptive and in an open state in order to feel the sensations and emotions arising out of the contact between himself and his partner. As the man remains in this state with his partner, orgasm can come without the vigorous movement that usually attends sexual intercourse. Most men who practice this often report a greatly enhanced sexual experience. Many couples do tantra who have never heard of pelvic pain.

Practicing tantra at first is not easy. As we have said, tantric practice requires a willingness on the part of the man to tolerate a sense of incompletion mixed with pleasure that comes from not rushing to orgasm. There are men who are not interested in exploring this practice and feel it is an intrusion upon their independence and freedom. Others resent having to practice such a level of impulse control. There are many men, however, who are in relationship with someone with vulvar pain who welcome any means by which to be sexually intimate. To be sure, even with tantra, most women with vulvar pain experience some degree of discomfort. This depends on what stage of dyspareunia they are in. Tantra, while having this limitation, still can help a woman who has vulvar pain enjoy sexual intimacy while minimizing what causes her pain.

Urethral syndrome and sexuality

If there is pain in the urethra upon touch, a woman can be in pain during intercourse as the penis pushes on the tender urethra. While these women are in treatment we sometimes recommend non-penetrative sexual activity as we have described above in relationship to women with vulvar pain.

Levator ani syndrome and sexuality

There is no known direct physical cause impacting or impairing sexual functioning in *levator ani syndrome*. As in other conditions where there is no physical cause impacting sexuality, sexuality tends to be affected whenever someone has pain.

Physical Exercise and Chronic Pelvic Pain Syndromes

The relationship between exercise and pelvic pain is not often addressed. There is little written about this subject even though many of our patients are anxious for advice about whether to initiate, continue, or stop physical exercise.

Some patients with prostatitis, interstitial cystitis and urethral syndrome have reported that certain kinds of exercise worsen their symptoms while other kinds do not. Others report that they feel better after exercise. Still others report that exercise has no effect on their symptoms.

Women with vulvar pain often report an increase in symptoms if exercise results in any kind of friction against or irritation of the vulva, including bicycling, horseback riding, sometimes swimming in highly chlorinated pools, or any kind of exercise in which the women wears tight clothing rubbing against the vulva.

In general, physical exercise lowers levels of anxiety and is beneficial for the body in numerous ways. Our general advice about physical exercise is that if you can find a form that does not exacerbate your symptoms, it is to be encouraged.

Physical exercise that aggravates your symptoms

Sometimes certain physical exercise is contraindicated. Patients who have enjoyed or benefited from these types of exercise ask us whether they should resume these exercises in spite of their increased pain, or whether they will ever be able to go back to them. Our view is that some kinds of physical exercise can aggravate pelvic pain because they put a strong demand on the pelvic muscles to contract—muscles which are already shortened due to chronic tension. These tensed, shortened muscles don't relax very well. When physical exercise tightens them further, they remain in an elevated state of tension for a while. For reasons upon which we can only speculate, some people's symptoms are affected while others are not.

The kinds of physical exercise that are most likely to aggravate symptoms of pelvic pain and dysfunction include weight lifting and body building as well as bicycling. We think that bicycling aggravates symptoms in some people because it pushes on the tender, painful trigger points in and near the perineum. These often highly trigger-pointed and tender areas are often not happy being pressed upon by bicycle seats.

Weight lifting and bodybuilding have been associated with the onset of pelvic pain in a number of patients we have seen. A few patients who undertook a crash course in flattening their stomachs reported that their pelvic pain began after their regimen of 500 sit-ups per day got into full swing. While all exercise causes a contraction of the pelvic muscles, sit-ups and weight lifting demanding the abdominal muscles to strongly contract, put a large burden on the pelvic muscles. It is not surprising that this kind of exercise can initiate or aggravate pelvic pain and dysfunction that arise from chronically contracted muscles.

There are doctors who insist that when the pudendal nerve is compressed, one must protect it by avoiding exercise like bicycling or rowing which tend to aggravate it. While pudendal nerve entrapment remains a controversial and speculative general explanation of chronic pelvic pain, if one is symptomatic, avoiding exercise like bicycling or rowing is a harmless precaution.

Hatha yoga and stretching

Part of our protocol in the physical therapy component of our treatment involves doing stretches to loosen the muscles in the pelvic floor that have been shortened. These are specific kinds of stretches aimed at assisting with the rehabilitation of the pelvic muscles and we include these exercises as part of our homework for the patient.

The muscles of the pelvic floor can be stretched to some limited degree. We believe the stretching that we describe in chapter 6 is the best way to use external stretches to lengthen and loosen contracted pelvic muscles. It is a kind of yoga.

Hatha yoga is an ancient Hindu practice of stretches that are called 'asanas' or postures, aimed at relaxing the body and preparing it for meditation. The popularity of yoga has grown in the west and in many places yoga studios are as common as copy shops or video rental stores. Hatha yoga receives our support as we see it helping the muscles to stretch and lengthen as well as helping the body to quiet. If there is a limitation of time, we encourage our patients to do the stretches described in this book that are specifically aimed at the lengthening and relaxation of the pelvic muscles.

While it is not part of our protocol, some patients have reported benefits from Bikram yoga which is a kind of yoga done in a hot room. The heat helps relax the body and may allow the muscles to be stretched more deeply. Bikram yoga or other hot room yogas tend to be strenuous and is not recommended for people with certain kinds of heart conditions or any other disorders or conditions that react adversely to heat and exercise.

Massage and body work

Whatever calms you and soothes you is good for pelvic pain. Full body massage, while sometimes costly and time consuming, is a very good activity for someone who has pelvic pain. Swedish massage, Shiatsu, Rolfing, Esalen massage, Jin Shin Jitsu, Reiki, Rosen Bodywork, Feldenkrais, Trager, Cranio Sacral Therapy, Tui Na, and reflexology, are all types of bodywork that usually have the effect of relaxation and quieting. While a number of our patients have unsuccessfully sought out these approaches as a primary treatment, we consider them useful in helping to establish a calmer state and saner life style.

Other Relevant Issues:Medications, Work, and Bladder Retraining

Medications for pelvic pain and dysfunction

We know of no curative medications for the kinds of pelvic pain and dysfunction described in this book. While there are generally no effective pain medications, there are some medications that can 'take the edge off' the pain on a temporary basis for some patients.

Antibiotics are sometimes successfully used for the very small number of cases of prostatitis categories I and II and IV. Estrogen creams are sometimes used to treat certain cases of *vulvodynia. nonbacterial prostatitis/CPPS), levator ani syndrome, proctalgia fugax, and urethral syndrome* are conditions for which doctors prescribe some medications. There are some medications that have varying degrees of success with interstitial cystitis.

In general there are no really effective medications to deal with the pain of chronic pelvic pain. Alpha blockers like Flomax®, Hytrin®, Cardura® and Uroxatrol® can offer some relief to some patients with pelvic pain, but there can be considerable side-effects for some patients including nasal stuffiness, elevated heart rate, and fatigue. Elavil®, originally used as an antidepressant, is sometimes prescribed in non-antidepressant doses for pelvic pain.

Perhaps of all the medications that have a limited efficacy for pain in the pelvis, the benzodiazepines like Valium® can help give the sufferer a 'break' from the pain. Sometimes patients will take 5 milligrams of Valium® every third day to help sleep, and in order to reduce the constant gnawing of the pain. Patients should exercise caution about addiction with these medications.

Narcotic medications

While there are a few exceptions, the patients with whom we have the least success are patients who regularly take narcotic medications. This isn't true of all patients who take narcotic medication as we have helped some patients to substantially reduce their pain and who are now free of taking such pharmaceuticals. In general, however, narcotic medications breed physical dependence, and in our view lower the pain threshold. The conditions we treat with our protocol seem somehow altered and less amenable to our treatment when affected by narcotic drugs.

Bladder retraining

When the pelvic muscles lengthen and loosen, it is sometimes helpful to address the habit of frequent urination that has developed when one was more symptomatic. The bladder receives about 1 cc of urine per minute. If the bladder has gotten into the habit of urinating frequently, and this persists even though symptoms have clearly improved, it is sometimes useful to change this habit by gradually postponing urination for up to an hour or two. This is done in small increments so long as such postponement is comfortable. In this kind of retraining, bladder capacity may be increased. This retraining should be done under the supervision of a physician.

If I am in pain, do I continue working or do I take time off?

There are advantages and disadvantages in holding down a full time job and functioning in every aspect of life while you are dealing with pelvic pain and dysfunction. The advantages are that you usually keep up your self-esteem by functioning fully in your life while you have symptoms. The obvious other advantages have to do with maintaining your reputation and financial stability, and keeping up with your obligations. Members of your family who rely on you are probably going to feel better knowing that you are continuing to function in a way that allows them to feel secure. The disadvantage of continuing to work exists when your work exacerbates your symptoms.

It is useful to consider the following questions with regard to working or taking time off. What best serves my recovery from my condition? What best serves my long-range goals in life? What best serves my self-esteem? What is the best course of action that I can take that allows me to be an inspiration to myself? If I were ninety-five years old and peacefully lying on my deathbed looking back at my life, what would I advise myself about what I should do now? There are few magic answers to these kinds of questions.

Why pelvic floor biofeedback is not a reliable indicator of the usefulness of our protocol

The following article was written by David Wise as a response to a question on the internet about the usefulness of pelvic floor biofeedback and has been included in this edition of *A Headache in the Pelvis*.

... I am responding to a request for a comment about the usefulness of intrapelvic biofeedback measurements in determining if pelvic pain is a tension disorder and appropriate for the Stanford protocol. My short answer is that electromyographic measurement of the anal sphincter with a biofeedback anal probe, used alone, is an unreliable measure of what is going on inside the pelvic floor. Unremarkable readings of the anal sphincter should not be used to rule out tension disorder prostatitis and pelvic pain or to dismiss the appropriateness of a treatment of the Stanford protocol.

Here is the longer answer. Let me say first that I have been a biofeedback supporter and practitioner for over 25 years. I had the best of training over many years from one of the luminaries of the field and have worked with many patients over the years with multimodal biofeedback for anxiety, functional cardiac disorders, and urinary incontinence among other problems. I continue to do neural feedback training with Steve Wall, one of the geniuses in the field of biofeedback and the designer of the remarkable biointegrator system. And I did biofeedback assessment and training in intrapelvic biofeedback at Stanford for a number of years with many patients.

I think that biofeedback that measures skin temperature, galvanic skin response, muscle tension, brain wave activity; respiratory sinus arrhythmia for problems other than pelvic pain is remarkable and enormously helpful. What I am saying below refers to pelvic floor biofeedback for prostatitis and chronic pelvic pain syndromes that we discuss in our book in which a sensor is inserted rectally or vaginally where readings are measured on an electromyograph. It does not refer to intrapelvic biofeedback for urinary incontinence which I happen to think is the best and safest treatment that exists for incontinence.

In my own case, when I was symptomatic, I did an hour or two of pelvic floor biofeedback on a daily basis for a year. After many months of diligent practice, my resting anal sphincter tone was a remarkable zero after about 15 minutes of relaxation. And I was very dismayed, like the person whose comment you sent to me, to find that I was still in pain at the moment that the anal probe registered zero. I was also disappointed as a clinician experienced in the successful use of biofeedback for other problems to find that the biofeedback measurement seemed to indicate (erroneously) that tension was not a central problem in my pelvic pain.

I didn't understand then what I understand now, which is that the electrical activity in the anal sphincter is, for the most part, the only area that the anal biofeedback sensor measures, and often says very little about what is going on with the other 20-some odd muscles within the pelvic floor. Furthermore, the biofeedback sensor measures dynamic muscle tension, but not chronically shortened tissue without elevated tone. It is possible to have a relaxed anal sphincter and have pelvic floor trigger points. In this case, elevated tone and active trigger points inside the pelvic floor are not reflected in the anal sphincter measurements.

Shortened, contracted tissue inside the pelvic floor, symptom-recreating trigger points when palpated and a tension-anxiety-pain cycle are the culprits in most people with pelvic pain that we successfully treat (which can sometimes includes a chronically tight anal sphincter as well in some) and we consider these factors criteria for diagnosis. For example, in my experience at Stanford, people with levator ani syndrome almost always have an entirely normal resting anal sphincter tone while palpating the painful trigger points on the levator ani muscle is excruciatingly painful. Resolving those trigger points and relaxing the inside of the pelvic floor can resolve this pain without much change in the measurement of the tone of the anal sphincter before or after treatment.

On our website, www.pelvicpainhelp.com, we have video clips of a important study, replicated many times, demonstrating that at rest, the electrical activity inside a trigger point in the trapezius, monitored by an a needle electromyographic electrode is quite high while the electrical activity of the tissue less than an inch away from the elevated electrical activity is essentially electrically silent. If you used a regular biofeedback sensor to measure the general tone of the trapezius, you may well find nothing remarkable and yet to rely on this information is entirely misleading and would incline you to miss the treatment that could substantially reduce or abate the pain and dysfunction coming from the active trigger point.

The bottom line here is that in my experience, electrical measurement of the anal sphincter, (or the opening of the vagina) used alone, is often poor measure of what is going on inside the pelvic floor. While I believe biofeedback is remarkably successful for many other disorders, and is one of the treatments of choice for urinary incontinence, vulvar pain, I am unimpressed with the usefulness of biofeedback in treating most male pelvic pain.

The best gauge of the usefulness of our protocol that treats pelvic pain of neuromuscular origin is a thorough examination of the pelvic floor for trigger points that recreate symptoms and palpating for tightened and restricted muscles inside the pelvic floor. This must be done by someone with a significant amount of experience in working with pelvic pain and with the kind of myofascial trigger point release that we use. An inexperienced person will miss all this and I have seen many times that even physical therapists who specialize in treating pelvic pain miss trigger points referring the symptoms to and inside the pelvis. This is one reason why we have offered trainings for physical therapists who treat male pelvic pain.

We sometimes find pelvic floor electromyography useful when there is a high pelvic floor resting tone, because it provides an objective marker that we can compare readings to after the patient has used our protocol. The idea that pelvic floor biofeedback measurements are a reliable test of whether pelvic pain is a tension disorder represents a misunderstanding of the problem and should not be relied on, especially when the readings are normal. Pelvic floor electromyographic measurement monitoring the anal sphincter is one of those medical tests where a positive finding may mean something and point toward the proper therapy and a negative result doesn't prove anything.

The Stanford Protocol and other manifestations of a headache in the pelvis: constipation, reduced urinary flow, bashful bladder syndrome, slow transit time, irritable bowel syndrome, anal fissures, and hemorrhoids

Chronic holding in the pelvic floor does not limit its manifestations to chronic pelvic pain syndromes. A modified Stanford Protocol may be useful in these consequences of chronic pelvic tension. These conditions include constipation, reduced urinary flow, bashful bladder syndrome, slow transit time, irritable bowel syndrome, anal fissures and hemorrhoids.

At some time or another, many people find a little blood in their stool, usually after a particularly hard bowel movement. One can become confused and upset at such an event. At other times, alarmed individuals go to the doctor complaining of rectal pain after a bowel movement with no apparent blood in the stool. Often the doctor gives the diagnosis of anal fissure or hemorrhoid to these complaints. Hemorrhoids constitute another condition that is painful and sometimes the source of blood in the stool. A hemorrhoid is a kind of varicose vein, which tends to balloon out when straining on the toilet.

One French study showed that one third of women had hemorrhoids or anal fissures after childbirth. One to ten million people in North America suffer from hemorrhoids. Both of these conditions are common in both men and women. These conditions are often related to constipation and diaharrrea. Constipation has been related to chronic tension in the pelvic muscles in adults and recently to refractory constipation in children in a study done at the Mayo clinic.

The colon and rectum are structures that operate together in the activity of the evacuation of stool. Normal, non constipative bowel function involves the reflex relaxation of the external anal sphincter and the pelvic floor muscles (along with sufficient tone in the colon) to allow the reflex sense of urgency with the filling of the rectum for fecal matter in the bowel to pass through the anal canal. Chronic tension in the bowel and pelvic floor triggered by anxiety can interrupt normal bowel function and can commonly result in constipation.

The anal fissure is like a paper cut in the anal sphincter. It is understood by many researchers that the anal fissure is called an 'ischemic ulcer.' Ischemia is a condition in which there is a significant reduction in blood flow to an area. The current understanding about anal fissures is that because there is elevated tension, the blood flow in the anal sphincter is reduced, thereby impairing the tissue which then becomes fragile and vulnerable to injury from a hard bowel movement or from the pressure of bearing down during defecation.

Diet has clearly been implicated in the development of the anal fissure. Cow milk consumption has been associated with chronic constipation and anal fissures in infants and children. Interestingly, a shorter duration of breastfeeding and early bottle-feeding of cow milk were also suspected to play a role in early incidences of anal fissures in infants and young children.

A Danish study showed a significant relationship between the absence of raw fruits, vegetables and whole grains and anal fissures. Furthermore, frequent consumption of white bread, sauces thickened with roux and bacon and sausages increased the risk of anal fissures. British researchers found that hemorrhoids and anal fissures were much more likely to occur when one did not eat breakfast.

While most anal fissures and hemorrhoids resolve themselves after they flare up, some colorectal surgeons lean toward a procedure or surgery to treat hemorrhoids and anal fissures. We have seen patients who are anxious about their rectal discomfort talked into an aggressive treatment of the fissure or hemorrhoid involving surgery.

It is generally agreed that the source of the anal fissure in large part involves a chronically tightened internal anal sphincter. Both surgery, the procedure of stretching or dilating the anal sphincter under anesthesia, and the application of topical agents to the internal anal sphincter are aimed at relaxing the anal sphincter. The surgical concept for anal fissures is based on the peculiar idea that cutting the sphincter is the best way to reduce the tone, tension and spasm in the anal sphincter. While surgery is often successful, there is risk of short term and sometimes long term fecal incontinence.

This conventional medical treatment of anal fissures, hemorrhoids and constipation tends to ignore the relationship between mind and body. Like the conventional treatment of prostatitis, the relationship of a person's mindset, level of relaxation during bowel movements, and management of stress is almost entirely ignored in the literature on the treatment of anal fissures. Instead, there is a narrow focus on immediately reducing symptoms of the anal sphincter, hemorrhoid or slow transit times involved in constipation. Procedures, surgery, laxatives and medications are the usual options for patients who suffer from these conditions. As with treatment of prostatitis, there is little literature on the connection or treatment of body and mind in the anal fissure, hemorrhoid or in problems of constipation.

The focus on a surgical intervention for the anal fissure or hemorrhoid is an expression of a viewpoint that sees no value and sees no intelligence in the symptoms someone with such a condition is experiencing. Instead of seeing an anal fissure, for example, as the way in which one's body is complaining of the diet, stress, bowel habits and anxiety one is under, conventional treatment sees the symptom of blood in the stool, rectal pain or abdominal pain as something that needs to be stopped. Little regard is shown for the big picture of a person's life and how one's symptoms are a response to this big picture. As we have said elsewhere, it is our view that the symptom is the way our bodies are trying to communicate. If we refuse to understand the message because we don't understand the body's language, we needlessly suffer and don't deal with the root problem prompting the symptom.

In the large majority of cases, it is the chronic tension in the pelvic floor, including the anal sphincter, usually combined with diet, and anxiety and time urgency around bowel habits that leads to anal fissures, hemorrhoids and constipation. The chronic pelvic tension, inappropriate diet, and bowel habits associated with most anal fissures, hemorrhoids and constipation do not come out of the blue. In a word, a person's mind and body and lifestyle are involved in the creation and perpetuation of these conditions.

Squatting vs. sitting during defecation as a way of helping the relaxation of the pelvic floor and benefiting individuals with a host of pelvic floor and colon related difficulties

Most people throughout history have squatted when they have evacuated their bowels.The modern toilet is relatively new in the history of mankind and has been adopted as the standard of a civilized bathroom appliance. The perennial hole in the ground over which one squatted to defecate is considered primitive in modern western society. A website (www.naturesplatform.com) devoted to promoting the advantages of squatting during defecation writes about the history of the modern toilet:

> "Human beings have always used the squatting position for elimination. Infants of every culture instinctively adopt this posture to relieve themselves. Although it may seem strange to someone who has spent his entire life deprived of the experience, this is the way the body was designed to function.

> The modern chair-like toilet, on the other hand, is a relatively recent innovation. It first became popular in Western Europe less than two centuries ago, largely by coincidence. Invented in England by a cabinet maker and a plumber, neither of whom had any knowledge of physiology, it was installed in the first dwellings to use indoor plumbing. The "porcelain throne" was quickly imitated, as the sitting posture seemed more "dignified" – more suited to aristocrats than the method used by the natives in the colonies.

> Two other influences also favored the adoption of this new water closet. One was the headlong rush to modernize all existing sanitation facilities (which were in fact non-existent). The public assumed that

all the benefits of modern plumbing required the use of the seat-like toilet, since it was the only one having the proper fittings to connect to the pipes. This assumption was incorrect, since toilets with all the same flushing capabilities could be (and have since been) designed to be used in the squatting position.

Secondly, in nineteenth-century Britain, any open discussion of this subject was considered most improper. Those who felt uncomfortable using a posture for evacuation that had nothing to do with human anatomy were forced to keep silent. How could they denounce the toilet used by Queen Victoria herself? Hers was gold-plated.

So, like the Emperor's New Clothes, the water closet was tacitly accepted. The general discomfort felt by the population was indicated by the popularity of "squatting stools" sold in the famous Harrods of London. These footstools elevated one's feet while in the sitting position to bring the knees closer to the chest – a crude attempt to imitate squatting.

The rest of Western Europe, as well as Australia and North America, did not want to appear less civilized than Great Britain, whose vast empire at the time made it the most powerful country on Earth. So, within a few decades, most of the industrialized world had adopted 'The Emperor's New Throne.'

A hundred and fifty years ago, no one could have predicted the effect of this change on the health of the population. But today, many physicians blame the modern commode for the high incidence of a number of serious diseases. Compared to the rest of the world, people in westernized countries have much higher rates of appendicitis, hemorrhoids, colon cancer, prostate cancer and inflammatory bowel disease."

There is compelling evidence that sitting on the toilet to evacuate the bowels is inferior to squatting in a number of ways. Squatting tends to relax the puborectalis muscle, which is essential in defecation. It tends to reduce or eliminate the need to strain and bear down to initiate defecation. A long study examining the effect of squatting during defecation and hemorrhoids showed improvement or elimination of hemorrhoids as the result of squatting during defecation. Doing the 'valsalva maneuver' in which one bears down to initiate defecation while holding one's breath has been sometimes associated with heart attack or episodes of atrial fibrillation because such a maneuver increases pressure in the thorax and interferes with venous blood returning to the heart. The heart rate can significantly drop during this activity. Defecating while squatting can reduce the need to bear down during defecation.

The modern toilet makes squatting during defecation problematic as it is made for sitting. Nevertheless, with a little innovation, it is possible to squat on a toilet. On www.naturesplatform.com a device is sold that allows one to easily squat during defecation. When pelvic pain also involves anal fissures, hemorrhoids or constipation, the issue of integrating squatting during defecation might well be considered.

We would like to see research on a non-invasive and self administered treatment of anal fissures and other headaches in the pelvis following a modified version of our protocol for pelvic pain. This may involve the rehabilitation of a tight pelvic floor using *Myofascial/Trigger Point Release*, modifying the habit of tightening the pelvic muscles habitually under stress using *Paradoxical Relaxation* and relaxing the pelvic floor while squatting on the toilet. While there is little research done on the treatment of these kinds of conditions using this perspective, we strongly support an independent study evaluating the efficacy of a modified Stanford Protocol including squatting on the toilet, for the treatment of constipation, reduced urinary flow, bashful bladder syndrome, slow transit time, irritable bowel syndrome, anal fissures, hemorrhoids, and other manifestations of headaches in the pelvis.

CHAPTER 8

STORIES OF PATIENTS IN
THEIR OWN WORDS

We have begun to collect stories from patients who have been trained in our protocol. We hope these accounts, in the patient's own words, can offer a flavor of what our treatment feels like as the patient and what is possible in terms of results from our program. Each patient below is writing after a certain amount of time of doing our protocol. We believe that the results can continue to improve as their skills at relaxation deepen.

Patient report after 2+ years of practicing protocol

In the summer of 1998 at the age of 21, I started to experience urinary frequency. It started out mild. In the mornings I would wake up to urinate and then lie back down in bed and not feel that I had completely emptied my bladder. I ignored it at first but after it persisted for a couple weeks I decided something must be wrong and went to see a urologist. He was unable to culture anything from my prostatic fluid, the extraction of which was the first of many uncomfortable and unnecessary procedures. He decided anyway that I must have a low-level infection of the prostate. I started taking antibiotics and it seemed to help initially–the first of a myriad of expensive and unnecessary medications which seemed to help the outset. Before I finished the medication the symptoms returned and after it was finished they remained.

The urologist was unable to provide any further recommendations. The next urologist I saw in December of 1998 had me pee into a uroflow device to measure my flow rate. He printed out a nice little graph to show me how my flow rate was lower than average and informed me that I had a urethral stricture which would require a dilation under general anesthesia and a prescription to Hytrin®. Anxious to be rid of my symptoms, I eagerly underwent the procedure. Improvement lasted only about 2 weeks.

When I called the urologist several weeks later to ask about my returning symptoms he instructed me to keep taking the Hytrin®, which I did for several months to no avail. My symptoms gradually worsened, but I did not experience any pain—only frequency.

I moved to San Francisco in August of 1999 and made an appointment to see a doctor at a prominent university whose specialties included chronic pelvic pain syndromes. He suggested that I might have interstitial cystitis and recommended I undergo a hydrodistention under general anesthesia to verify this. In February of 2000 I underwent the procedure and the results were uncertain. It was a "soft call" as to whether I had IC. I definitely lacked classic IC symptoms (no pain, no prominent food sensitivities) but the doctor could think of nothing else it was likely to be.

Soon I began a cycle of trying out new medications, becoming excited that they were working at first and then quickly becoming disappointed as my symptoms returned and remained. The frequency gradually became worse than it had ever been before, but still it was only frequency and not pain. There was some extremely uncomfortable frequency at times (bathroom visits 15-20 times a day and 4-6 times a night) but nothing I would describe as pain ever manifested. Also at this time I was beginning a new job which was significantly stressful. In retrospect I think this was a major factor in the worsening of my symptoms, along with a spiral of hopelessness as each new medicine I tried failed to help. I tried the usual battery of meds that is prescribed for IC and after 6 months when it seemed they were not working at all I began to try other things such as numerous over-the-counter herbs, additional prescription antibiotics of different types, the hypertension drug Amlodipine®, etc. etc.

I estimate I tried 20-25 different medicines or products over the life of my symptoms, none of which helped me to any significant degree. I tried transcutaneous electrical nerve stimulation. I underwent two urodynamic evaluations at two universities (both requiring catheterization while awake) and there were no remarkable insights gleaned from either study. I spent countless hours combing the internet and the university medical library for some additional scrap of information that might prove useful.

Eventually I stumbled onto an article written by David Wise on www.prostatitis.org called "The New Theory of Prostatitis as a Tension Disorder." I contacted David and since he was in my area I went to see him in November of 2000. I made some half-hearted attempts to start the relaxation therapy at home but didn't really begin it in earnest until early January, 2001. It was very difficult to sit through an entire tape at first and I squirmed and fidgeted throughout most of the tape. The therapy certainly teaches you patience. At this time I also began seeing a physical therapist recommended by David who specializes in CPPS.

With the combination of relaxation twice a day and physical therapy once a week I slowly began to see some steady improvement in my frequency over many weeks' time. It was always the case that I felt better for a day or two and then felt worse again for a stretch of days, but over time the good days began to outweigh the bad. The good days that I did have were the best days that I'd experienced in over a year.

These days were extremely encouraging and the memory of them is what carried me through the bad stretches, although after many bad days in a row it was often easy to think that I had been fooling myself.

When a good stretch occurred, though, it seemed unmistakable that my symptoms were improving. I had many good stretches that occurred with increasing frequency throughout March, April, and May, and by June '01 for the first time since they had begun I felt that I had a solid handle on my symptoms—that I was on the sure path to healing myself completely. I would definitely become cocky at times and stop doing the relaxation or stretches. My symptoms would not immediately return but if I persisted in a chronic state of stress for some time without paying attention to what was going on in my pelvis then they would creep back and suddenly demand my attention. In fact I can still say that this is the case—that I experience low-level symptoms from time to time but they are not something I fear anymore because I understand the factors that lead to their appearance and the factors that lead to their abatement. In addition, the intensity is very, very minor compared to what it was at the height of my misery. When symptoms do occur they are so subtle that they hardly enter my consciousness and I experience myself as having completely normal bladder behavior.

I practice the formal relaxation less frequently now (2-5 times a week depending on how things are going) and my pelvis seems to be perfectly happy with that. I live my life in a more relaxed state overall and that makes all the difference.

I consider myself lucky when I read other peoples' accounts of their experiences with CPPS. However I would not hesitate at all to describe my own experience as a waking nightmare. I remember in the midst of it coming home from work exhausted and collapsing onto my couch in tears, not sure if I could hold down my job, if I would have to move back home with my mother, etc. My social life was severely impacted. I skipped countless activities on account of how uncomfortable I felt and because I dreaded having to go to the bathroom every 30 minutes in public. I didn't date for 3 years. I sunk further and further into misery and desperation and I believe my symptoms would have continued to worsen had I not found David's article online.

The relaxation techniques were a godsend for me. They have helped me in more ways than in just the abatement of my symptoms. I feel more centered now, more at peace in general. In one way of looking at it I can consider my symptoms to have been a gift, because they are the only thing that could have led me to devote so much of my time to the relaxation, which in retrospect I desperately needed though I have never thought of myself as an uptight person. I have never battled with depression except as a result of my symptoms. I have only experienced mild anxiety from time to time and always as a result of outside circumstances. However I believe now that I am genetically predisposed to holding the tension that I do feel in my pelvic muscles. I say it's a genetic predisposition because of the fact of my maternal grandfather's identical symptoms and the existence of bladder problems in general on my mom's side of the family.

A metaphor I have found useful is that one's pain can be like a compass —it's trying to lead you to where you need to be. The story of my own struggle has in a sense been the story of learning to read my personal compass and to trust it and check in with it every now and then, with the goal of not having to check in with it at all because I am following it all the time without effort. When I was physically suffering it's like the compass was shoved in my face and I would get really gung-ho about the relaxation. When the symptoms abated I started to wander off the path, but like I said this was necessary for learning. Now the compass is much clearer to me even when I'm not suffering and I can detect the path intuitively.

In sum, I suffered from prostatitis/CPPS for three years and my life became absolutely miserable. I received four different diagnoses from four urologists, tried over 20 prescription medications, vitamins, and herbs, and underwent several very uncomfortable and expensive procedures, all of which did hardly anything to help my symptoms which had slowly been increasing in intensity over time. Using the protocol described in *A Headache in the Pelvis*, I slowly I began to heal myself, without any medication. Six months later my symptoms were diminished significantly and nine months later I felt I was healed. It is now 2-1/2 years after I first started to practice these methods and I feel that I have been freed of this horrific condition.

There are many schools of thought regarding this syndrome and I studied all of them obsessively at one time. I feel very strongly however that over the coming years the ideas in this book will eclipse the other models of this disease and come to be recognized as the most powerful methods for dealing with it as more and more people are seen to have solid and long-lasting benefits. Mine is not the last testimonial you will see. I should say however that it is not a simple or quick solution and it requires a lot of devotion, but chances are the end-result will be your freedom. My advice to those who are still suffering is "best of luck; do not abandon hope until you have given these methods your most sincere effort."

Patient report after practicing protocol for 8 months

I am a 35 year-old male who, until recently, suffered from chronic prostatitis for over 15 years. I am writing to share my experience in hope that someone else currently suffering from my predicament can heal as I have.

Starting at about age 18, I began to notice symptoms of high urinary frequency and a great sense of urgency when I felt the need to urinate. By the time I was 24, the symptoms reached the point where I was uncomfortable much of the day. I went to see multiple doctors, including several urologists who did several invasive procedures. I had diagnoses that ranged from chronic prostatitis to a narrow bladder neck. Other than taking alpha-blockers, doctors told me they could not do much to help me.

I somehow learned to get by with my symptoms. I always sat on the aisle row of a movie theater or airplane to facilitate my many visits to the restroom. I would map out the restrooms first upon entering a new mall or other unfamiliar place. I tried to avoid any event where I would not be assured access to a restroom hourly. I typically felt the urge to urinate every hour during the day. Multiple visits to the restroom at night were not uncommon. I budgeted more time to sleep because the quality of my sleep was so poor.

In October of 2002, the inconvenient and annoying symptoms of my condition turned into a persistent pain. Urinating no longer relieved, even temporarily, the pain and sense of urgency to urinate. I felt pain in and around my urethra, my bladder, and my prostate. Multiple visits to several urologists resulted in a diagnosis of "chronic prostatitis." I started taking any pharmaceutical that the doctors suggested, including antibiotics, alpha-blockers, Ambien® to sleep at night, muscle relaxants, and anti-inflammatory drugs. None of these helped. By Thanksgiving, I wasn't able to sleep more than a few hours per night. I began missing work. I spent entire days in tears. I suffered from panic attacks. I went to the emergency room. I started to avoid people as much as possible. My increasing anxiety made the pain even worse.

I can remember thinking in December, 2002 that everything I had spent my whole life trying to achieve was coming to an end. I had an MBA from Harvard Business School. I had a great job. I had a loving wife and two children. I had a strong relationship with God. Yet, I couldn't see how I was going to survive. I didn't see how I could possibly maintain my job with this pain. I didn't even think I would be able to enjoy watching my children grow older. Sex was out of the question because it just exacerbated the symptoms. I would have gladly given up all my money and material possessions to be cured of the acute pain that plagued my every moment.

In desperation, I turned to the internet. Fortunately, I learned about the work of Dr. Wise and Dr. Anderson. Contrary to many other approaches I read about on the internet, their approach appealed to me because:

1. It had a fundamental basis. In other words, it made sense that the pain I was feeling was the result of constriction of the pelvic region.
2. It did not entail pharmaceuticals or surgery. Surgery is permanent. Pharmaceuticals were not working and had bad side-effects. I was intent on not resorting to narcotics of any kind.
3. Their approach allowed me to be proactive about my pain. Some internet sites claim that chronic prostatitis is caused by an as-yet unidentified and untreatable infection. What good would it have done me to convince myself that I had an untreatable infection?
4. The symptoms I felt and the way I felt them matched those described in *A Headache in the Pelvis*.
5. My symptoms historically have been linked to stress. Having increased tension in the pelvis during times of stress seemed to fit my profile as well.

My wife drove me to San Francisco to start therapy. I first saw a urologist who ruled out other possibilities and confirmed that I might benefit from this course of therapy. I attended daily physical therapy with a therapist trained in the techniques. In addition to internal stretching performed by the therapist, I was put on a program to stretch various muscles and fascia daily. I began learning "moment-to-moment" relaxation. I also began learning and practicing the *Paradoxical Relaxation* technique. Within a week, I was much better. My wife drove me home to Los Angeles, where I continued physical therapy twice a week and later once a week for about three months. I became better and better at "moment-to-moment" relaxation of the pelvic muscles, to the point that I didn't need to think about relaxing those muscles any more. I continue daily *Paradoxical Relaxation* using tapes provided by Dr. Wise. Amazingly, the pain has diminished with each week that has passed. While there are occasional flare-ups the general trend was and continues to be in one direction–better.

It has now been eight months since I started this program. I have had to dedicate significant time to this effort. However, I feel like a miracle has been granted to me. My urinary frequency has dropped to only once per night and once per two hours, at most, during the day. I feel little, if any, pain. I feel almost no pain following sex. I am better than I have been in over 15 years!

Patient recovery with no physical therapy or formal relaxation training

While most patients require both *Paradoxical Relaxation* training and intrapelvic *Myofascial/Trigger Point Release*, we have received numerous emails from people reporting that their symptoms improved after the reading of our book and of hearing of a possible solution to their difficulty. Here is the story of a patient like this.

I first experienced prostatitis when I was around 23 years of age. Basically, I developed a rather noticeable pain in my left groin that simply irked the heck out of me and would not go away. Numerous urologists diagnosed it as epididymitis, but the funny thing was that it wasn't particularly responsive to the antibiotics that were prescribed. Moreover, it had this rather strange tendency to occasionally migrate to the right side, in which case the strong pain I had felt on the left would totally vanish. For about a year, it manifested primarily on the right side. Then, it switched back to the left. The discomfort generally didn't go away, though over time, what initially felt like a pretty distinct pain in my scrotum generally became a more generalized feeling of discomfort. It stuck with me throughout my graduate studies. Even during my first professional job in an office, it was there, without any sign of relief. Basically, it not only irritated me but also worried me tremendously.

After about eight years, I had pretty much resigned myself to living with that condition indefinitely, which was not a rosy picture at all. Luckily, by that time, the internet had taken off as a vital source of medical information. After reviewing numerous websites, I came across the findings of Dr. Wise. I was struck by two things. The first was the startlingly accurate description of my condition in his writings. It seemed he had a handle on what was going on, which was namely that this "condition" seemed to be in a category all its own. The second thing was the real breakthrough: the possibility that the ultimate source of this discomfort was not any infection, not any structural abnormality, but simply TENSION, muscular tightness that restricted the entire area that was affected.

To make a long story short, this basic insight was nothing less than a breakthrough for me. I eagerly contacted Dr. Wise, to learn as much as I could about his "theories." I was always pleased to see that his model of prostatitis seemed to accurately reflect all the rather subtle qualities of this strange condition with which I had been living. For example, I noticed that my discomfort would increase dramatically whenever I had caffeine, or whenever I became stressed over anything. Perhaps the most important discovery offered by Dr. Wise was the knowledge that this condition had its origin ultimately in my own state of mind, or mental state of dis-ease. As such, I knew I myself could fix it, simply by "unwinding" so to speak.

Within about a six month period after simply learning about what was really going on, I basically found the symptoms disappearing. In other words, simply realizing that my own thoughts and beliefs were at the root of this proved to be the best medicine. Simply by refusing to worry and, even simply by just understanding my condition, miraculously, the pain went away! Now of course, this does not mean there was no effort involved, or that it happened overnight. But the one thing that is clear is this: the less helpless I felt towards my situation, the more it improved.

Basically, the first step was just plain knowing that "nothing was wrong," and the second step was making a concerted effort to relax and work through and accept the pain, even when it was still there. By learning to see the pain as acceptable, so to speak, I managed to put it out of mind. Once I had gotten into a pattern of really being able to stop thinking about it (which is much easier once you know it has no real "physical" basis, at least not in the form of a virus), it just plain vanished! Basically, I am now free of prostatitis.

Patient report after practicing protocol for 2 years

In October of 2000 I had a vasectomy performed by a urologist in Toronto. Before the operation I inquired about its safety and the possibility of side effects. I was told the operation was routine and there was no possibility of any problems. In June of 2001, I began to experience severe pains in my testicles. These pains were severe enough to force me to give up employment. For several months I was unable to do much more than stay in bed. In addition to the pain I was unable to ejaculate. I saw a urologist at Mt. Sinai Hospital in Toronto who recommended a vasectomy reversal. It was scheduled, but as the pain spread from the testicles to the perineum and the entire pelvic area, my urologist felt that the reversal might do more harm than good.

He instead put me under the care of the pain clinic at the hospital. I was given large doses of opiates, 36 mg of hydromorphine contin per day, which lessened the pain but did nothing for the underlying condition. In November 2001 I came upon your article, "The New Theory That Prostatitis is a Tension Disorder." I spoke to Dr. Wise a number of times on the phone and in December 2001 went to California. I was seen by Dr. Rodney Anderson, urologist and Tim Sawyer, physiotherapist. My wife accompanied me on the visit and learned the technique of myofascial release inside the pelvic floor from Tim Sawyer.

At first my wife was unable to perform the internal massage because it was too painful, but after a month of external massaging, she was gradually able to do the internal work. She did this twice a week for about two months. It gradually became easier to do and eventually the frequency of the massages was much reduced. At the same time, I began daily relaxation exercises, using a course on tape. I also did various stretches recommended by Tim Sawyer.

The pain grew gradually less severe during 2002 and I gradually reduced the number of grams of painkiller I was taking. By the late months of 2002 I was taking only one mg. per day. Since January 2003 I have taken no painkillers on a regular basis. I visited Dr. Wise and Tim Sawyer again in March 2003. Tim was able to confirm a significant loosening inside the pelvic floor. I continue to feel some pain every day but rarely is the pain severe enough to take any opiate. The degree of pain from day to day varies a great deal.

Some days are entirely pain-free except for occasional discomfort in the pelvic area; some days involve pain for longer periods and more intensely. There is usually some pain during and after sexual intercourse, but ejaculations are normal. I occasionally use aspirin or ibuprofen. In general I would say I'm pain-free about three-quarters to seven-eighths of the time. For the other quarter or eighth the pain is present but bearable.

For a long while I was taking a drug called Imovane to help me sleep at night. I discontinued the Imovane about a month ago, but I am now frequently awakened by the need to urinate during the night, which is a disturbing problem. I have been advised to try Flomax, which I used at the height of the problem but discontinued about a year ago.

The relaxation exercises, myofascial release, and stretches seem to have helped me reduce my pain very significantly. Although I am not back at a full-time job I have been able to work part-time as a consultant and university lecturer. The alleviation of the pain has of course made life much more worth living for me. I am grateful for your patient and understanding help.

Patient report after 4 years of practicing protocol

Beginning in about 1992 (age 27), I experienced occasional pelvic pain, primarily the right side in an area stretching from my groin and extending upward. It was a dull ache. I am a military lawyer. I saw a civilian urologist who conducted a thorough pelvic and prostate exam and concluded there was nothing wrong with me (except a small, benign, and unremarkable spermatocele resting on the top of the right testicle). He examined my prostate fluid under a microscope with negative results. The pelvic pain was worse just above and to the right of the pubic bone and in the lower abdominal area.

When I was stationed overseas from 1994-1996, the pain became progressively worse. I tended to usually have a dull ache in the pelvis just above the pubic bone and to the right. The pain was worse if I had to stand for a long time (e.g. in a courtroom or on a subway). I got to where I would want to sit down and "rest" to relieve the ache, even though I was physically fit and not tired. I didn't want to walk anywhere. In concert with the pelvic pain, I experienced pain that would radiate down my right inner leg and back thigh and rear, sometimes as far down my leg as the calf.

Another symptom was that my urine flow was typically very, very slow. It would sometimes slow to an intermittent trickle, and I learned that if I took a deep breathe and exhaled while standing at the urinal, the flow rate would accelerate a bit. Usually, it took me a long time to urinate, and after going, my bladder still felt full. I remember during some of my first court trials in 1995, I had an intense urge to urinate, even after I just went, and it would feel as though I had to urinate virtually the entire day. During this time I started feeling an occasional, sudden, sharp pain somewhere inside the rectum. This pain would last for up to 10 seconds and would slowly release on its own. It was sometimes so intense and sharp that I was seized with pain and couldn't move until it subsided. (Imagine a severe toe cramp in your rectum). The pelvic pain level would fluctuate from between 0 to 4 or 5 on a scale of 10, and it was usually between a 1 to 3.

In addition to the pelvic pain, the pain in the inside thigh, and slow urination, I usually also felt a tight feeling in the area between the testicles and rectum for about an hour after sex, as though the path for the sperm had been tightened or blocked. In 1996, I moved to the West Coast, and these symptoms continued.

I went to several military urologists, both overseas and in California, who diagnosed me with chronic prostatitis. In 1997 I experienced these symptoms on and off. In 1998, the symptoms became worse. I was prescribed Ciprofloxin® 500 for about 75 days for chronic prostatitis. The doctors never found any evidence of a microbe infection in my prostate fluid. One doctor also inserted a lighted camera into my urethra and examined the path leading up to my kidneys and bladder—all tissue was healthy. After the antibiotics and tests, I still had an aching pelvis, and was still "double eliminating" (on the advice of one of the doctors, urinating 10 minutes after I urinated in order to try to make the bladder fully empty). My side ached nearly all the time and no one knew why.

Fortunately, the military urologist had heard a paper delivered by Dr. Rodney Anderson at a conference on prostate massage. The urologist thought Dr. Anderson might be able to help me, so he referred me to Stanford Medical Center. Dr. Anderson did a complete physical examination. That exam found the unremarkable spermatocele, but more importantly, some "pressure points" of pain. Dr. Anderson sent me immediately to see Dr. David Wise.

When I first began the treatment I was skeptical; I could not believe that my pain was unwittingly a self-inflicted wound. After I learned to be conscious of my body, and to reflect on the holding and tightness in my pelvis and the pain I felt, I became convinced. It took some time— months, and I cannot recall when I crossed the line, but I became absolutely certain that my symptoms were relieved by the protocol.

Over the course of my year of training in progressive (paradoxical) relaxation, I learned to totally relax my mind and body. When I received myofascial release therapy from a physical therapist prescribed by

Dr. Wise, I could actually feel when the tension inside was released by stretching the tissue; it was instant and soothing relief when a "tight" spot was stretched. It got to where I could feel where the pressure point was and could direct the therapist to it quickly. My wife has also been trained in the myofascial release therapy, and she occasionally treated me in 1999 and early 2000, but stopped after the pain subsided. She stands willing to continue that protocol if the pain flares-up.

In the last four years, I have integrated this relaxation method into my life. Each day, I practice momentary relaxation and the deep relaxation, stretching (taught by the physical therapist), and breathing in concert with relaxation. I try to make time for one complete session of progressive (paradoxical) relaxation session each day, but in my current position I cannot always do so.

At the present time, I do a complete session of 45-55 minutes 2-3 times per week, and a shorter session of 15-25 minutes on all other days. I also practice conscious effortlessness throughout the day by relaxing the pelvis, and practice contractions, and stretches, which were taught by the physical therapist. I also do a continuous, almost subconscious series of checks throughout the day to search for and release any tightness and holding in my body, particularly in my pelvis and the sides of my face. When I practice relaxing my body, my head and neck become so relaxed that my head bobs gently and unconsciously with the flow of the blood to the head. As a result of this relaxation, the blood vessels in my body relax and widen, and after a few minutes, my hands and feet become flush with blood.

Because of my military job and lack of privacy in Washington, D.C., I have adapted and learned to practice a full session of progressive (paradoxical) relaxation while lying with my head on a towel in the building gym—with a loud game of basketball taking place on the court next to me, or while laying on the sidewalk or grass as planes landing at National Airport roar overhead. These conditions are not ideal for relaxation, but it does work well. Because I have been taught to effectively abandon effort, I can focus on my breathe and heart beat rather than the noise. I don't fight or stress about the noise around me, but just let it be there as I drift away. I have done the same thing on a ship—with bells clanging and announcements being made over the loudspeaker. I have learned to be profoundly relaxed.

Usually I have no pelvic pain. Rarely, when I am stressed or busy at work, I feel a low level ache. It is usually nonexistent, but will fairly rarely be present at a low level if I become very stressed or busy at work. This stands in stark contrast to before I began the protocol when the pain was there all the time and occasionally severe.

One of the most important benefits is that I am certain of the source of the pain, conscious of the feeling and aware of the tendency to subconsciously tighten or hold the pelvis. I now feel how I tighten (and can focus on releasing) the tension. I am also aware of how the level of pain is linked to the pace of stress in my life. One more thing: until I wrote this, I had forgotten the emotional and mental worry, and fear that I had over what was mysterious pain and symptoms. Now I feel I am in control, the worry and fear have vanished. I know the recipe for getting well—discipline for exercising daily relaxation.

Until I wrote this I had also forgotten the slow urine flow that I used to have—standing at a urinal taking as long as four or five other men to urinate. My urine flow is now strong. I had also forgotten how I always had the feeling that I had to urinate soon after I already went. Now, I have a feeling of a totally empty and comfortable bladder. The discomfort after sex has now abated except for rare instances—it now occurs about twice a year. This treatment and protocol has changed my life.

Patient report after five years of practicing protocol

In late September of 1997, two years after retiring, I started having problems with urination. Some brownish colored "sediment" started showing up at the end of urination and then pelvic pain started. My pain was in the rectum and prostate areas. When I woke up in the morning there was generally no pain, but it built up during the day and was worst in the evenings. My internist prescribed an antibiotic and referred me to a urologist. The urologist prescribed traditional treatment for prostate infection including antibiotic and ibuprofen. After six weeks of treatment virtually no progress was made. I observed during this period that pain killers provided no relief but muscle relaxants did help. Naps on the floor were the only other thing that seemed to help.

The symptoms were ruining my life and at times I was depressed. I was losing weight and there didn't seem to be any light at the end of the tunnel.

A close friend got me an appointment in mid-December 1997 with Dr. Tom Stamey, the pioneer of urology who was still at Stanford. Dr. Stamey determined in one hour that I had no evidence of infection in the prostate gland and referred me to Dr. Anderson and Dr. Wise. I had no idea what form of treatment they would provide.

Dr. Anderson had me see a physical therapist that specialized in myofascial pelvic floor muscle pain relief. He relieved "trigger points" in various pelvic floor muscles and even taught the procedure to my wife who happens to also be a PT. I bought medical textbooks on myofascial pain and read extensively about the subject.

Dr. Wise started to teach me *Paradoxical Relaxation*. Gradually I started to make progress. One of the difficulties is that progress is an up and down process. I remember several times getting discouraged and phoning Dr. Wise. His calm, steady, reassurance was very helpful. One day, a few months after starting his therapy I asked him how long it would take to perfect his technique. He hesitated for a while but finally said "about two years."

After two months I had made enough progress to know that things were on the right track. Oddly, knowing it might take two years was encouraging as I knew what to expect and not to think that I would be all cured in a month. My progress steadily got better and after a year I was 80% better. After two years I felt like I had reduced my symptoms by 90%.

It is now about five years since I first started treatment with Drs. Anderson and Wise. I feel that my symptoms are 99% gone but more important I know how to deal with symptoms if they occur. Happily, I seldom think about the problem any more.

CHAPTER 9

MORE THAN YOU EVER WANTED TO KNOW ABOUT THE MEDICAL SCIENCE OF CHRONIC PELVIC PAIN

In this third edition of our book we wanted to attempt an update of what is happening on a national level to investigate and understand the problem of chronic pelvic pain syndrome (CPPS). There are many individual physicians and medical centers who take a special interest in this problem and the plight of those suffering from it. The National Institutes of Health has received a directive from the Congress to pursue effective treatment modalities for CPPS and, through a consortium of awarded medical centers (UPPCRN), is making significant progress in this endeavor. Meanwhile much effort needs to be exerted to figure out how the condition starts and then evolves to become the significant life-altering malady that it is.

CPPS is a non-malignant pain perceived to be occurring in structures associated with the pelvis. There are no gold-standard objective tests that define CPPS. No one can verify and quantify the amount and intensity of pain. Only a few stalwart physicians and scientists have endeavored to uncover the possible biologic basis for its existence and to attempt any kind of rational medical treatment. Although there are *more than two million office visits a year in the United States for complaints about prostatitis,* and variations of this disorder make up almost 10% of a typical urologist's practice, they are not the most welcomed of patients and complaints because there are no definitive therapies to help these patients. In this chapter we will review many of the scientific studies and publications devoted to characterizing and managing chronic pelvic pain syndromes.

If one looks at the history of medicine, the pelvic malady of *prostatitis was only first described in the middle of the 19th century.* Imagine all those men suffering for centuries without a clue as to what might have been going on. In the first part of the 20th century someone introduced the theory of a possible role of bacteria and examined prostatic fluid microscopically. The secretion was cultured for the first time in 1913. It was not until 1968, however, that Dr. Thomas Stamey and Dr. Edwin Meares at Stanford University established an appropriate, detailed patient examination that allowed the urologist to document scientifically that bacteria were truly originating from the prostate gland and not the urethra or the urinary bladder.

The anatomy: organs, nerves, and muscles

Our problem with CPPS centers on identifying the anatomical parts of the pelvis that actually cause the pain. Of course all pain transmits through *sensory receptors, then into pelvic fine webs of nerves culminating in the spinal cord and, ultimately, forwarded to the brain* where it is perceived subjectively in different ways and interpreted by each patient. Physicians traditionally assign *blame for pain to the various organs of the pelvis.* Reproductive organs such as the uterus, the vagina, the testicles, the penis, the prostate gland, and excretory organs such as the rectum and urinary bladder, receive this blame. We typically attribute pain to these organs rather than suspecting the supportive structures of these organs (nerves, ligaments, and muscles). It is difficult to understand the dull and diffuse nature of pelvic pain unless you understand how nerves work, and that there can be communication between nerves (cross-talk) as well as intermingling of signals that can confuse someone about where the pain is really originating. There is also the phenomenon known as "referral" whereby pain coming from an organ can be felt in more remote areas including the skin. Because of the intimate relationship between the nerves, a strong signal from one area may stimulate a neighboring nerve, even though that neighbor nerve was not being irritated by the stimulus. This may represent the method whereby muscles become tense that is not related to the source of irritation. *There are 27 different muscles and a panoply shrub of nerves in and around the pelvis* associated with the bony structures and organs. These structures obviously play an indispensable role in association with the organs they support.

As the myriad of nerves interlace throughout the pelvis, the stimulating nerves responsible for smooth muscle contraction and organ function, as well as motor nerves that control supporting muscles, balance and complement each other. We divide muscles into smooth muscle and striated muscle. Smooth muscles exist in the walls of the intestines and provide the motility of our intestinal function; similarly the urinary bladder, the uterus, the ejaculatory ducts, the prostate and even the heart is functioning with a type of smooth muscle. Our skeletal or striated muscles are responsible for voluntary movements and offer support to the pelvic structures. Adrenaline, in the form of a biochemical called norepinephrine, stimulates smooth muscle through the adrenaline receptors embedded in the muscles. These receptors *are extremely sensitive to small amounts of this substance.* We designate these smooth muscle receptors as alpha- and beta-receptors. The heart is full of beta receptors, for example, and when one is excited, even mentally, adrenaline causes the heart to go into a racing configuration. The smooth muscles in the pelvis, while confined primarily to the organs, respond in the same way to mental signals that release adrenaline and cause a reaction in the pelvic muscles. There are also adrenaline receptors in the contracting or striated muscles of the pelvis that can be excited by release of excitatory biochemical substances—these are responsible for the "fight and flight" response that gives us extra energy. This is why people can sometimes perform heroic maneuvers in stressful situations.

Dr. Steven Kaplan and colleagues at Columbia University reported that the inappropriate contraction of the external urinary sphincter during voiding can be misdiagnosed as chronic prostatitis. An interesting observation in their review included the fact that 91% of the subjects in this study were firstborn sons. Dr. Kaplan's group felt that behavioral modification and biofeedback to teach the appropriate relaxation approach to urinating was a good therapeutic option.

Chronic prostatitis as the model of pelvic pain in men

Chronic prostatitis means different things to patients and doctors. It is a common diagnosis, but clearly a misnomer. There are three cardinal symptoms associated with the diagnosis of chronic prostatitis—pelvic pain and discomfort, disturbances in urination, and abnormal sexual function. *The primary symptomatic complaint that becomes chronic is pain or discomfort.* It is important to understand the circumstances at the time of onset, how long and cyclic the discomfort has been occurring, and what degree of intensity is involved, and where the pain is located. We also evaluate the patient's attitude towards his pain, whether the pain is variable or constant, and if he/she is having pain-free intervals.

The second set of symptoms includes *disturbance of urination*; typically a sense of urinary urgency and frequency, inhibition of the ability to release the urine, a burning sensation or "dysuria" with voiding, and depressed flow. There may be dribbling of urine at the end of emptying the bladder because of poor balance between the sphincter muscles and the contraction of the bladder, often resulting in "trapping" of urine within the urethra as it runs through the prostate.

The third set of symptoms is *disturbance in sexual function* that may include loss of libido or sex drive, inability to attain erection, or to maintain erection for satisfying sexual intercourse and, most importantly, discomfort with ejaculation. Sometimes there can be a spasm-like discomfort immediately after ejaculation or a discomfort that lasts as a nagging annoyance for several hours or days. There may be changes in the spermatic fluid such as decrease in volume, blood staining on occasion, and watery or clumpy discolored semen.

The physician's exam

When physicians examine a patient they typically focus on the organs of the pelvis; they perform a rectal or vaginal examination and attempt to palpate the uterus, the prostate, the bladder, testicles, etc. but usually *ignore the important integration of the muscles and the fascia or ligaments holding these organs.* It is our considered view that when evaluating a patient with chronic pelvic pain it is imperative to do a thorough evaluation of the muscles and ligaments surrounding these organs. It is our duty to elicit with the examination what the patient experiences and attempt to correlate what we find with any possible abnormality that may be occurring either in the organs or in the pelvic muscles. This is not a simple task. The majority of patients suffering with chronic pelvic pain have no classic standard findings that can be easily detected. There are however, certain basic urologic evaluations that should be done including a careful medical history and documentation by questionnaire of the patient's perception of his problem.

In our *evaluation at Stanford*, as do most urologists, we *examine the prostate for microorganisms and inflammatory white blood cells.* Typically this requires the patient to urinate a small amount prior to examination, to compare this sample microscopically to what may be found in voided urine after massage of the prostate. We palpate the pelvic muscles looking for actual trigger points or specific discomfort zones, especially surrounding the prostate. We then feel the prostate gland itself. We determine its consistency, whether it is soft or "boggy", whether there are areas of induration or hardness—this may represent fibrosis or scarring from previous inflammation—but we must remain ever vigilant for cancer. Checking muscles and tender points, we methodically massage the prostate gland, beginning at the base and milking it toward the center on each side to express prostatic fluid into the urethra. The prostate is composed of 20-30 small microscopic tunnels (acini) emanating from the periphery of the prostate. Each glandular unit is connected to the outside world by a tiny duct that opens into the urethra on each side of the main ejaculatory duct located in the center of the prostate. These tiny ducts expel the enzyme-rich prostatic secretion with prostate contractions at the time of sexual ejaculation.

The easiest way to perform this pelvic examination is with the patient lying supine with the legs spread in stirrups. This allows the examiner to have leverage and direct visualization of the penis and the urethral opening to be able to collect prostatic fluid. We have found it convenient to collect the fluid with a tiny sterile glass pipette, the prostatic secretion drops accumulating with capillary action as they appear at the penis opening or meatus, particularly when there are only one or two drops that are quite precious to be able to examine and culture.

Once the prostatic fluid has been collected, the patient will urinate a small volume to provide a washout of prostatic fluid that can be separated, analyzed and submitted for bacterial culture. This is particularly important when no prostatic fluid is expressed out. We advise patients to refrain from any sexual ejaculation for seven days prior to coming in for the examination to afford a better opportunity to maximize collection of prostatic fluid. Older men typically have more prostatic fluid because the gland is larger as it increases in size with age. Younger men find it a challenge to refrain from sex for a week.

We take the patient's prostatic fluid to our office laboratory where a simple examination under the microscope (after staining the fluid with a dye) helps identify white cells and improves the analysis. We count the number of white cells in the prostatic fluid to compare with counts from normal, asymptomatic men and to track changes as a treatment program is instituted. This detail of performing careful analysis of the prostatic fluid is usually conducted only in academic or university medical centers where an intellectual curiosity prevails. Unfortunately, quantifying the degree of inflammation from massaged ducts has failed to yield any correlation with patient symptoms. This relationship between pain and inflammation is poorly understood.

Imaging of the prostate in chronic prostatitis

The best way to look at the prostate gland tissue is to use transrectal ultrasound (TRUS). It has not gained wide acceptance as a method of evaluation but can often be quite valuable in demonstrating inflamed tissue, the presence of stones in the ducts (representing urinary mineral deposits), swelling and thickening of seminal vesicles (semen storage organs behind the prostate) and accurate measurement of the size of the gland.

Japanese investigators have used computerized x-ray images and angiography or dye in blood vessels to evaluate chronic pelvic pain. They demonstrated excellent three dimensional graphic images of veins around the prostate. There existed considerable congestion in these veins behind the bladder and along the sides of the prostate in patients suffering with pain. The veins on the surface of the prostate were much thicker in diameter than in subjects with no pain. This basically represents varicose veins of the prostate. This is suggestive of heightened tension in the muscles of the pelvic floor and is supportive of our view that chronic pelvic pain syndromes are associated with muscle tension.

It is quite common for urologists to look inside the urethra, prostate and bladder in patients suffering from this disorder with a technique called *cystoscopy*. This consists of passing a pencil-sized flexible probe with magnifying optical lenses, high intensity fiberoptic light, and associated video camera up the penile urethra. *However, cystoscopy may be the least productive procedure that can be done.* Some urologists will say to the patient "Oh, yes, I see some inflammation in the prostate." This is anatomically impossible because they are only looking at the surface of the urethra and not at the prostatic tissue itself. There is rarely, if ever, any obvious inflammation on the surface of the prostatic urethra in the condition of prostatitis.

Urodynamics

One investigative tool to evaluate urinary and prostate function consists of physiological measurements with a procedure called *urodynamics*. This diagnostic procedure evaluates physiologic function of the related smooth and striated muscle function in the bladder, prostate, and external sphincter. This testing consists of placing a small pressure-sensing catheter in the bladder to detect changes in bladder pressure; the catheter can simultaneously monitor the urethral voluntary sphincter pressure activity and associated pelvic floor function. An important component of this testing consists of placing a catheter balloon in the rectum to monitor abdominal pressure. We utilize electrical sensors patched to the skin around the anal muscles to detect electrical activity within the pelvic floor, both with relaxation and voluntary contraction, but primarily to determine how much relaxation is achieved when attempting to urinate.

Most of the work devoted to evaluating the pelvic floor and looking at the muscles of the pelvis has focused on urinary incontinence in women. In this situation there is an obvious loss of muscular control needed to maintain the urinary bladder as a reservoir-coughing, laughing and sudden movements cause urinary incontinence. While this is an important medical dilemma, the concept of precisely how this happens has been controversial and it remains a focus of attention by most clinicians, mainly gynecologists and urologists, because it represents a lucrative surgical opportunity to fix it. It is now important for us to shift our attention to the pelvic floor and to the complex interaction of the muscles within and around the organs of the pelvis as a basis for evaluating chronic pelvic pain.

While urologists are trained surgeons, surgical procedures have failed to offer any solution to the chronic pelvic pain syndromes we discuss in this book. It is the hope of the authors that urologists will carefully consider complementary methods of patient care, especially in relationship to chronic pelvic pain. At the same time, medical practice guidelines should be evidence-based and not advocated solely on *opinions* of efficacy. As previously described, well-educated patients and patient advocates are seeking greater control of their treatment and the planning thereof by focusing on preventative maintenance issues and partnering with physicians in their disorder management.

How common is infectious prostatitis?

Acute bacterial prostatitis, as described earlier, is a *fairly easy diagnosis to make*. It is associated with pain in the prostate, difficulty urinating, high fever, chills and weakness. It is serious because bacteria can spread into the blood stream causing sepsis or blood poisoning. Acute bacterial prostatitis requires aggressive antimicrobial therapy and sometimes needs catheter drainage of the urinary tract. Inadequately treated acute bacterial prostatitis may potentially become dormant and develop into recurrent chronic bacterial prostatitis. We typically treat acute prostatitis for a total of 28 days using potent antibiotics. We administer antibiotics for about 6 weeks when chronic bacterial infection is established.

There has been great debate about whether chronic pelvic pain represents an infectious disease? *The consensus of expert opinion today is that chronic prostatitis, as a medical disorder, is probably caused directly by microbial agents in only about 5% of the cases.* Most of these episodes of bacterial prostatitis are without symptoms between infection flare-ups. Men who complain of chronic pelvic pain and who have been diagnosed with prostatitis may possess increased bacterial counts found in the prostatic fluid. *But the bacteria are normal flora, or normal types of bacteria in the urethra, and they colonize the prostate ducts in low numbers just as we find normal resident bacteria in the vagina, the mouth, the rectum, and other parts of the body.* Uropathogens, however, are bacteria not normally found in the genitourinary (GU) tract and are known to be invasive and cause inflammation of both the prostate and bladder. These bacteria are organisms from the intestinal tract. When a physician identifies significant numbers of these bacteria in the genitourinary system, either in the urethra, the bladder, or coming from the prostate gland itself, he or she considers this to be bacterial cause of the symptoms. Are we not trying hard enough to find poorly detected microorganisms that may be responsible for inciting this condition? Some have suggested we should culture the body fluids for a longer time to detect the slow-growing bacteria that may also be hiding out under biofilms. There is evidence that the bacteria were there as sleuthed out using DNA tracking. It appears that those individuals who suffer from CPPS do indeed have a higher incidence of the positive DNA fingerprints when you take biopsies from their prostates compared to men who never had CPPS.

Serious investigators have looked at multiple microorganisms that might be the cause of chronic prostatitis, including microbe forms such as *Chlamydia, Ureaplasma,* and even parasites or protozoans such as *Trichomonas. While very small percentages (3-10%) of patients have been found to carry these unusual organisms, there have never been convincing studies to prove that these organisms are specific causative agents.* Dr. Andrew Doble and associates from England performed an exhaustive search for infectious agents in chronic prostatitis syndromes using ultrasound-guided tissue biopsies of the prostate.They found that 88% of their patients had chronic inflammation in the tissue, but only 15% of patients had any organisms that were cultured or grew from the tissue, and actually these were considered to be contaminants from the skin. *This information again reinforces the concept that we are dealing with a painful disorder and no proven microorganism as a cause. Unfortunately, most physicians and patients believe chronic prostatitis to be an infectious entity and are searching for the Holy Grail of antimicrobial treatment that will once and for all eradicate these pesky organisms from their system. We believe this is a fruitless quest.*

Another controversy that continues to be debated among urologists and microbiologists is whether *gram positive organisms* (a laboratory stain classification) such as *Staphylococcus saprophiticus,* or *Staphyloccocus epidermidis* and *beta strep,* commonly found as normal flora in the urethra, may indeed act as pathogenic bacteria or organisms that would invade and cause inflammation. These gram-positive microbes are usually found on the skin and in the mouth, as opposed to gram- negative microbes that come from the large intestine. While some patients may have large numbers of these organisms in the urethra and colonizing the prostate, use of antimicrobials to eradicate the organisms does not *seem to provide improvement in symptoms and there is very little association with the cause and effect of symptoms.*

Dr. Wolfgang Weidner from the University of Giessen in Germany has been an important contributor to evaluating the occurrence of microorganisms and inflammation in CPPS. He published a paper in 1991 demonstrating a thorough search for microorganisms in hundreds of consecutive patients. He found high numbers of bacteria and several sub-bacterial species of *Ureaplasma* in a typical prostatitis pattern associated with increased numbers of white cells in the prostatic secretion. At that time he felt there was an important difference in the classification between patients with and without inflammation in the prostatic fluid, and that there were differences in the symptoms from those patients that had no white cells and pain in the prostate (the NIH classification difference between IIIA and IIIB). Our own anecdotal experience suggests a difference between the two categories in symptoms and in response to therapy. *We believe that patients who have no inflammation seem to have more neuromuscular dysfunction, more myofascial trigger points, and respond more rapidly to the Myofascial/Trigger Point Release and Paradoxical Relaxation. However, a careful NIH-sponsored study concluded that there is no correlation between evidence of infection or inflammation in the prostate and the symptoms of prostatitis/chronic pelvic pain. The precise relationship of prostate inflammation and chronic pelvic pain remains to be elucidated.*

The inflammation debate

In the first place we have only small shreds of evidence that inflammation may be involved in causing the pain of CPPS. Even less well understood is what biologic or physical entity may be inciting the inflammation. In a few instances some tissue has been available for sampling—bladder, prostate, rectum, vagina—and no obvious microbiologic substance appears to be an initiator. Furthermore, the presence and degree of inflammation does not correlate quantitatively with the degree of pain.

We have referred to the NIH study in which it was clearly found that no relationship exists between infection/inflammation and severity of pain and dysfunction in prostatitis. The occurrence of infection/ inflammation in chronic prostatitis/CPPS fails to be consistent and not always helpful in diagnostic terms. Dr. John McNeal, a devoted research pathologist at Stanford University, has worked on prostate disease, particularly prostate cancer, his whole professional life; he found many years ago that between 5-15% *of men over the age of 60 have inflammation in their prostate tissue on microscopic examination but absolutely no complaint of pelvic pain.*

Doctors determine that there is inflammation in the prostate ducts when they look at expressed prostatic secretion under the microscope at 400 times magnification. However, it is not always possible to massage prostatic fluid from a patient. We then must rely on a post-massage voided urine specimen and separate prostatic fluid by centrifugation from the urine for analysis. Anecdotally, our male patients with prostatitis who have high numbers of inflammatory white cells in their expressed prostatic secretion actually seem to have less pain on average than those with few or no white blood cells coming from the ducts of the prostate.

As we do not have documentation of infectious agents causing chronic pelvic pain syndrome, the unanswered question remains; what is causing the inflammation? Many investigators believe that it has to do with *dysfunction of the voiding* mechanism, an imbalance in the urinary muscle control causing reflux or pressure of urine and hence toxic substances of urine backing up into the prostate gland ducts creating an inflammatory and irritated condition. In simple language, tension in the pelvic muscles may be inhibiting the free flow of urine, causing it to back up into the prostate. This backed up urine, in our view, may then cause the mild inflammation that is found in approximately 1/3 of patients with a diagnosis of prostatitis.

Dr. Linda Shortliffe, a urologist at Stanford, performed an analysis of the prostatic fluid proteins in an attempt to look at differences between men with bacterial and nonbacterial prostatitis. She had previously established that patients, even with nonbacterial prostatitis, could have elevated levels of prostatic immunoglobulins. Contrary to popular thought, this paper demonstrated that bacterial prostatitis and nonbacterial prostatitis had significantly lower levels of PSA compared to those with pain only, or those who were uninfected.

In 1995, Dr. Robert Nadler reported the effect of inflammation on PSA levels. The presence of inflammation was quite common, and nearly all of the men with high PSA levels had a least one biopsy specimen positive for chronic inflammation. Confusing the issue, however, 77% of those with normal PSA levels also had foci of inflammation on biopsy. In many cases, acute and chronic inflammation was more prevalent in the high PSA group that was at 63%, versus 27% in the normal PSA group. They concluded that a quantitative demonstration of acute and chronic inflammation in the tissue was not necessarily associated with clinical bacterial prostatitis, or even symptoms, but may be an important contributor to elevated PSA levels in the blood.

More recent investigations of a possible immune response with nerve growth factors and associated inflammatory agents known as cytokines raise some intriguing possibilities. Firstly, it may reveal biological markers that could be analyzed to show an abnormal presence and provide potential therapeutic blocking agents for the inflammatory condition. It has been shown that very small amounts of nerve growth factor, perhaps released because of primary prostate nerve damage, can increase sensitivity to both thermal and mechanical stimulation. These kinds of chemical changes may be related to altered sensitivity to pain and be responsible for the dynamics of fluctuation in this chronic pain syndrome.

Not finding an elusive inflammatory inciting agent or evidence of obvious inflammation does not detract from our belief and supporting evidence that the central nervous system—the brain and spinal cord—in conjunction with powerful immune regulating mechanisms known as the hypothalamus-pituitary-adrenal (HPA) axis may be intimately involved in altering inflammatory events in the body related to CPPS. Neurogenic inflammation is a phenomenon that has been demonstrated in experimental models. It is clear that the autonomic nervous system, particularly the adrenergic or sympathetic system plays a very important role. Sensory nerve endings are activated and they then release biochemicals known as cytokines and a myriad of other inflammatory mediators, which in turn affect the surrounding tissue. Small microvessels dilate and become more permeable, increased blood flow (causing redness) and exuding blood plasma allows white blood cells to accumulate. This is acute inflammation. This inflammatory process often, in turn, excites or activates the stress system, causing anxiety and recycling the neurogenic inflammation. The hallmark of chronic inflammation is infiltration of tissue with mononuclear inflammatory cells ("mononuclear cells", "round cells", i.e., monocytes, lymphocytes, and/or plasma cells). Generally, good tissue has been (and is being) destroyed, and there will be some evidence of healing (scarring, fibroblast proliferation, angioblast proliferation). We believe that distress (emotion)-related immune dysregulation may be one core mechanism behind a large and diverse set of health risks associated with negative emotions. This field has been labeled with such terms as *Psychoneuroimmunology* and *Psychoneuroendocrinology*.

This book unfortunately cannot serve as the forum to expound on the multiple scientific studies that show these relationships and pathophysiologic phenomena. We must, however, always hold our beliefs in abeyance and begin thinking, remaining open minded about the possibilities in our quest to understand this CPPS malady.

Muscle tension and chronic prostatitis

Because we have so little to go on in documenting a cause of chronic pelvic pain, theories and partial bits of evidence are discussed interminably. Clearly, evidence-based treatment is needed but multimodal shotgun therapy still prevails. Fortunately, new concepts and efforts are being expended to unravel the mechanisms involved and to examine the interface between pain and inflammation, and between the nervous system and the immune system. The NIH, through the NIDDK branch, is providing funding for cooperative investigation and we hope this gathering of the minds will bear fruit.

Some key pioneer clinician-investigators attempted to evaluate the neurophysiology of the pelvic floor and its relationship to chronic pelvic pain. Drs. Dirk H. Zermann, Manabu Ishigooka, Ragi Doggweiler and Richard A. Schmidt at the University of Colorado in Denver, showed that in men with chronic pelvic pain there was a strong association with neuromuscular and myofascial (muscles and ligaments) dysfunction. In a clinical evaluation of 103 patients seen at their clinic, 91 men (88.3%) had abnormal tenderness of the striated or voluntary muscle of the pelvis, and this myofascial tenderness was virtually always associated with inability to relax the pelvic floor efficiently.

Diane Hetrick, a physiotherapist, and the team with Dr. Richard Berger at the University of Washington in Seattle have recently confirmed the opinion that musculoskeletal dysfunction occurs in men with chronic pelvic pain syndrome. A higher percent of increased pelvic floor muscle tone, pain with internal palpation, increased tension with external palpation, and pain with external palpation were found in patients with CPPS as compared to healthy controls. Furthermore, these investigators at Washington showed that there exists hypersensitivity in the pelvic (perineal) sensory nerves of patients. They used a flash heat technique to create a painful heat stimulus in the perineum. When compared to healthy volunteers there was definitely more sensitivity to the heat pain in those patients suffering from chronic pelvic pain syndrome. Now we just need to figure out what mechanism is responsible for inducing and maintaining this pain in order to treat it specifically.

Some physician specialists (rheumatologists/immunologists) working with arthritis believe that the primary abnormality leading to expression of symptoms in fibromyalgia and related conditions consists of errant central nervous system function. This concept promotes the idea that there may be skeletal muscle abnormalities in patients having pain. It appears that a generalized disturbance in the pain perception threshold and the tension phenomenon from the central nervous system underlie these disorders.

Neuromuscular imbalance, or dysfunction in voiding, continues to be a prominent suspect of causation in chronic prostatitis. This certainly fits our model of tension myalgia and chronic pelvic pain syndromes leading to imbalance in urinary function causing inflammation in the prostate. A study published in 1987 by Dr. Wayne Hellstrom and colleagues from the University of California, San Francisco, promoted this concept with case reports. Their physiologic studies revealed elevated urethral pressures where the urinary channel runs through the middle of the prostate, causing reflux of urine minerals and toxic metabolites into the peripheral or outer zone of the prostate, the location of most of the inflammation. The peripheral zone ducts are perpendicular to the course of the urethra and certainly would be susceptible to high pressure in the prostate. Specific measurements of intra-prostatic pressure have been undertaken in patients suffering from chronic prostate pain, and in a series of 42 patients were found to be significantly elevated in a majority of them.

Dr. George Barbalias from Greece has also been a proponent of this mechanistic cause of chronic prostatitis. He was one of the early advocates of using potent alpha receptor blockade as a method of treatment. He utilized needle electrodes to actually measure electrical signals from the external urethral sphincter. He found normal motor unit potentials in the majority of the patients and discovered that there was a coordinated function of the detrusor and the external sphincter during the voiding. He noted that there was no difference between inflammatory and non-inflammatory patients, but that both groups had a decrease in their urinary flow rate. He described this as a *functional* urethral obstruction but not an actual physical obstruction. This *functional* urethral obstruction may well be the result of chronic pelvic muscle tension.

For many years *investigators felt that an imbalance in the urination pattern was a fundamental cause of inflammatory prostatitis.* In 1984 some investigators showed that 50 patients with a diagnosis of chronic prostatitis had abnormal urinary behavior. They found that 23 of those 50 patients had overactive bladder, with a hypersensitivity or "trigger-happy" bladder contraction occurring frequently. Similarly, in these patients they described evidence of obstruction at the bladder neck or in the prostate with high pressure voiding. They noted increased external sphincter muscle zone pressures, particularly during voiding. Some investigators believe elements of urethral obstruction to be of paramount importance in this condition. The urethral opening at the tip of the penis may be constricted. This may cause just enough backpressure for urine to reflux into the prostatic ducts.

Stress stimuli and the prostate

Throughout the years, many physicians and clinicians have been impressed with the *features of stress and/or anxiety contributing to pelvic pain syndromes.* In 1986 a group from Sweden (Lars Gatenbeck) studied rats that were stimulated and stressed with or without hormone additives. They investigated the microscopic changes of the prostate under these conditions. Inflammation of the gland was thought to occur because of stress reactions increasing output of adrenaline and other biochemical neurotransmitters. There was also a purposeful evaluation of any decrease in prostatic blood flow that could result in an inflammatory reaction and changes in the tissue. In their experiments, rats were submitted to stress stimuli for ten days. Examination of the prostate tissue after this kind of activity demonstrated moderate infiltration of inflammatory cells—there was a significant difference in those rats that received stimulation and those that did not, the latter having little or no inflammation. At the same time, they found a reduced serum testosterone level, but it was not clear what the influence or importance of this hormonal change could be. The other feature that was noted was that the lobes of the rat prostate having the least advanced drainage system had a greater involvement in inflammatory manifestation. Measurements of blood flow showed that the rat prostates had decreased blood flow during the experimental stress stimulation. This is an example of one of the very few experimental attempts to document the behavioral effects on both physiologic and microscopic changes. *It would not be a difficult leap of imagination to transfer this to the human condition and understand the effects of stressors and anxiety that could be contributing to the chronic pelvic pain syndrome.*

Another pivotal study of stress as a factor causing clinical prostatitis emerged in 1988. Dr. Harry C. Miller studied 218 men who had complaints typical of chronic prostatitis. Sixty percent or 134 of these patients were followed carefully, and their management consisted only of stress control. *With this psychological approach alone, 86% reported that they were better, much better, or cured. Most importantly, repeat cultures, prostatic massages, instrumentation, and medications were not utilized at all in this group of patients as he relied solely on stress management.*

Treatments and current national trial

The National Institutes of Health have been extremely interested in promoting clinical research regarding the pervasive disorder of chronic prostatitis and chronic pelvic pain syndrome. They are obviously most interested in finding a satisfactory treatment. A recent nationwide study evaluated the two most common medication treatments for the disorder: oral Ciprofloxin (Cipro®), a potent fluoroquinolone antibiotic and/or oral tamsulosin (Flomax®), a potent alpha nerve receptor blocking agent for the smooth muscle of the prostate and urethra. These two pharmacologic agents were tested in a blinded fashion against a placebo or sugar pill as a treatment of these syndromes. This is an important study because no one has ever systematically evaluated the effect of antibiotics on these "nonbacterial" disorders, although many doctors and patients claim improvement. The outcome of this study showed that the symptom scores improved slightly regardless of whether the patients took the antibiotic, the alpha blocker or the placebo. The contribution of an alpha-blocking smooth muscle relaxant continues to be debated with regard to its efficacy. In our own practice, virtually every patient who comes to see us has been previously treated either with potent antibiotics and/or alpha blocking agents, but they continue to have recurrent complaints.

Dr. Daniel Shoskes recently investigated the use of a dietary supplement known as a bioflavonoid. Quercetin was given to patients with chronic prostatitis/CPPS in a blinded fashion for one month. Patients taking the substance had their symptom scores decrease from 21 to 13 (67% improvement). This therapy seems to be well tolerated and offers significant symptomatic improvement in many men with chronic pelvic pain syndrome.

Heat therapy of the prostate

While heat therapy (hyperthermia) is not an approach we advocate, some studies have reported favorable results. Thermal therapy consists of various forms of heat induction—microwave, radiofrequency, laser, and ultrasound energy—where in place of 'cutting' tissue as in surgery, the prostate tissue is heated to a temperature that may cause tissue destruction. A publication in 1993 described 54 patients who had significant prostatitis symptoms for a period of over two years despite several courses of antimicrobial or anti-inflammatory therapy with no significant clinical benefit. The method of treatment utilized transrectal hyperthermia and the target temperature was only 42.5°C, therefore not creating any significant damage of tissue. Transrectal ultrasound was used to detect changes in the prostate volume or shape after the procedure. Overall, 50% of the patients reported an improvement in the quality of life; 47% reported no change. *This would be consistent with a strong placebo effect.*

In 1994 Dr. Curtis Nickel reported using transurethral microwave thermal therapy at higher temperatures ranging from 45-60°C that do cause death of prostatic tissue. Patients with nonbacterial prostatitis showed significant reductions in their symptom severity indices; 47% had a marked improvement at three months. However, this *again is not far from what one would expect from a simple placebo effect* but it also has the attendant considerable risks associated with inserting a microwave device in the prostate and destroying prostate tissue.

Prostatic massage with Myofascial/Trigger Point Release

Prostatic massage has been utilized by several generations of urologists, particularly prior to the advent of antibiotics. In a report from a Philippine study, repeated prostatic massages revealed occult organisms. This study has received much attention and popularity. Therapeutic benefit from massage may derive from expression of ductal acini contents that were not being emptied. This treatment may diminish prostatic pressure. The frequency of prostatic massage seems best when done twice weekly.

Dr. Daniel Shoskes has proposed massage plus antibiotic treatment. His patients underwent prostatic massage plus antibiotics for 2 to 8 weeks and 40% had complete resolution of symptoms, 20% had significant improvements, and 40% had no improvement. There was no correlation between inflammatory content and bacterial cultures.

Our opinion as expressed in a review article from *Techniques in Urology*, Vol. 5, pg 1, 1999, favors repetitive massage of the prostate, not for emptying the gland, but rather to relieve pelvic tension and release myofascial trigger points. *We continue to be extremely skeptical of the concept of occult bacteria that needs to be "massaged out." A simple analysis of repeated prostate massage is a "blind approach" to treating the disorder, wherein occasionally the right trigger point or myofascial source is appropriately touched.*

There is emerging interest in utilizing behavioral pelvic floor rehabilitation techniques in treating male CPPS. A group from Northwestern University Medical School in Chicago promotes the use of biofeedback in pelvic floor re-education as well as bladder training for this disorder. They recognize that pelvic floor tension myalgia contributes to the symptoms. They looked at a small group of 19 men, average age of 36 years, and treated them with this non-interventional process. The men showed improvement, particularly in their urinary scores, but also had a significant decrease in their median pain scores, from 5 to 1 on a scale of 0 (no symptoms) to 10 (worse symptoms). This is a preliminary study, but it confirms that a formalized neuromuscular re-education of the pelvic floor muscles benefits these patients.

We are not the first doctors to have considered the kind of treatment we are describing in this book. As early as 1934 there were a few physicians who understood that pelvic pain is related to tension or spasm of the pelvic muscles. George Thiele, M.D. was a proctologist (now referred to as a colorectal surgeon), who developed a physical treatment for pelvic pain that he generally included under the name coccygynia (pain of the coccyx or tail bone). Thiele's findings were later confirmed by Shapiro in 1937 who referred to pain around the coccyx as the Thiele Syndrome. In an article in 1963, Thiele reported on 324 patients who had pelvic pain in and around the rectum and anus. He, along with several other researchers, recognized that coccygectomy (surgical removal of the tail bone) failed to help anyone with pelvic pain other than those who had severe trauma to the tailbone. Furthermore, he acknowledged that there was no evidence of any disease of the coccyx or adjacent areas.

Thiele's contribution of applied massage to the levator ani and coccygeus muscles yielded remarkably good results. In some papers in the colorectal studies that followed, his treatment was referred to as Thiele Massage. He reported that over 90% of people that he treated improved after such treatment. He was a pioneer in this area, and while he published his results for doctors in his field to consider, somehow his work has disappeared and is rarely referred to in the literature on pelvic pain. The reason for this may be both economic and ideological. There is little economic incentive for colorectal surgeons to do Thiele Massage. Furthermore, colorectal surgery indicated by its very name, tends to be surgical, and massage of the pelvic muscles may not be seen as a good use of the surgeon's time.

Mehrsheed Sinaki, M.D. was a physician at the Mayo Clinic in the department of physical medicine and rehabilitation throughout most of the 1970's. Doctor Sinaki reviewed the medical records of patients who had a diagnosis of pelvic pain in general, but at that time more often referred to by the terms piriformis syndrome, coccygodynia, levator ani spasm syndrome, proctalgia fugax, or simply rectal pain. Absent were reports of urinary symptoms or of diagnoses including prostatitis, interstitial cystitis, or some of the other conditions we include in this book. This important article documented that the treatment that yielded the best results in these patients was as discussed earlier, the Thiele Massage. Sinaki acknowledged that the conditions he examined were obscured by many vague and chronic complaints. Furthermore, he found, as we find today, that a general medical exam and routine laboratory and x-ray exam are unremarkable. He wrote:

"The neurologist finds no neurological abnormalities and the orthopedist usually finds no bone, disk, bursa, or tendon …hemorrhoids or fissures may be inadequate (to diagnose the problem) because the levator ani, coccygeus and piriformis muscles and their attachments are often not carefully palpated."

Sinaki believed that the definitive test for the conditions he was reviewing was the digital-rectal examination in which the doctor inserts his finger into the rectum to feel the state of the muscles. He observed, however, that the normal digital-rectal examination was inadequate to assess the tenderness of the muscles.

Segura and other colleagues of Sinaki at Mayo Clinic reiterated Sinaki ideas in the Journal of Urology in 1979. They wrote:

"Patients with symptoms suggestive of prostatitis or prostatosis who do not have pathogenic bacteria in the prostatic secretions may in fact not have prostatic problems. The possibility of pelvic floor tension myalgia should be considered."

Drs. Hubbard and Berkoff, Department of Neurosciences at the University of California, San Diego, discovered that trigger points, which we usually find inside the pelvic floor of our patients, show spontaneous electrical activity. Travell and Simons, who introduced the concept of trigger points and myofascial release, defined the standard by which trigger points could be identified. Those standards were as follows:

1. Palpable and firm areas of muscle, usually referred to as *the taut band*

2. In the taut band, a little spot of great tenderness and sensitivity, especially upon the use of manual pressure

3. A pattern of sensation involving pain, sometimes in combination with tingling or numbness when this area is palpated digitally

4. What has been called a local twitch of this spot of tautness when the trigger point is pressed

Until the time of this study, trigger points could only be identified with a finger and there was no objective measure of the trigger point itself. The fact that trigger points could only be identified by individual palpation and not by objective measures left open the significance, and even the reality of the trigger points. In this important study, an objective measure of trigger points was found.

Hubbard and Berkoff placed needle electrodes in the trigger points of the subjects of their study. They also placed needle electrodes immediately beside the trigger point. They connected the needle electrodes to an electromyograph (EMG), which is a very sensitive machine for measuring electrical activity. Electrical activity in muscle is considered to be a measure of its level of activity.

Their results were remarkable because they found a sustained level of increased electrical activity in the trigger point, while there was no increased electrical activity found in the tissue immediately beside the trigger point. They theorized that this prolonged increase in electrical activity becomes painful by affecting the spindle capsule. (The spindle capsule is a microscopic part of the muscle tissue that the authors speculated was affected by the increased electrical activity and was the source of pain). This increased electrical activity was seen to be associated with the pain experienced subjectively, either when the trigger point is pressed on or even when it is not.

We have found the presence of trigger points in a large majority of our patients who have pelvic pain and dysfunction. We often (not always) are able to recreate the symptoms of patients we see when we press on these trigger points. We also find that when we complete a course of myofascial treatment, the trigger points usually disappear along with the pain and exquisite sensitivity. Furthermore, the reduction of trigger point sensitivity is often directly related to a subjective improvement in patient symptoms. The findings in this study, in confirming objective and measurable activity specifically within the trigger point, as well as our own clinical experience offer compelling evidence that the trigger points found in the pelvic floor are likely to have central significance to a person's experience of pain in other chronic pelvic pain syndromes.

Kruse and Christiansen examined the temperature of the skin in the area to which pain was referred after a trigger point was palpated. This study provides some objective basis for validating patients' reports of referred pain from a trigger point. They found that the area where a patient reported referred pain had a colder temperature than adjacent skin areas. It is assumed that the colder area is caused by a reduction in blood flow. Therefore, the area of referred pain being colder than the adjacent tissue supports the idea that ischemia (reduced blood flow) may be part of the pain and dysfunction we see in patients who have chronic pelvic pain syndrome.

In a conversation with Dr. Richard Gevirtz, who has done research in the relationship between trigger points and emotional reactivity, he shared with us that the impetus for the research that discovered increased electrical activity in trigger points in relationship to stress or anxiety originally came from Italian researchers and their work in the early and mid 1990s. They had claimed that indeed the sympathetic nervous system activity directly affected skeletal muscle and particularly the spindle part of the muscle.

Gevirtz and Hubbard showed in the mid 1990s that trigger point activity significantly increased when the subject experienced anxiety, and the trigger point activity significantly decreased in the absence of emotional arousal. Needle electrodes monitored electrical activity in trigger points of subjects asked to do arithmetic calculations (a standard way in which researchers arouse anxiety). In considering the results of this study that connect anxiety and trigger point activity, we can begin to make sense of the intimate relationship between stress and pelvic pain and dysfunction symptoms reported to us by many of our patients.

In our own work, we routinely have measured the level of muscle tension in the rectum and the vagina of patients who come to see us for pelvic pain and dysfunction. Men with prostatitis had an increased level of pelvic floor muscle tension. This level was reduced after they participated in the treatment program that has led to the current one.

Dr. Howard Glazer at Cornell University in New York, in a personal communication, reported that men who had prostatodynia had higher than normal levels of rectal tension and that their resting level of tension was what he called "unstable" compared to normal subjects. Furthermore, he found that the level of strength in the contraction of those muscles of the prostatodynia patients was higher, but more unsteady than normal.

Glazer has consistently seen increased levels of vaginal tension in women who have vulvar pain. He also typically sees a weakness in the strength of contraction of these women when they are asked to do Kegel exercises monitored by an electromyograph. The focus of Glazer's successful approach with women with vulvar pain has been to help them relax, strengthen, and stabilize their pelvic muscles.

Pudendal nerve entrapment

We need to mention the concept of the pudendal nerves being compressed or entrapped in the pelvis as a potential cause of chronic pelvic pain. Surgical procedures have been developed to release ligaments of the pelvis and to transpose nerves away from these impinging structures. Patients with this syndrome typically have considerable pain while sitting that is completely relieved when standing. It is also considerably relieved by sitting on a toilet seat. There are theories that athletic endeavors may have caused distortion in the nerve pathway. Similarly, chronic constipation may contribute to the condition.

Several nerve injection studies to document the source and relief of pain are necessary before any surgery is undertaken. Certainly, any surgical approach to alleviate this condition must rely on documentation of nerve dysfunction as measured by nerve conduction studies. It appears that less than 50% of patients are successfully relieved of their pain with surgery. We believe our myofascial release therapy may provide significant relief before surgery is considered.

Isolated male orchalgia (pain in the testicles)

Chronic orchalgia, or pain in the testis, vexes a lot of young men and they reluctantly bring this to the attention of their physician. Testicular pain occurs most commonly in young men in their 20's and 30's and requires careful history and physical examination, because this is also the age group where testicular cancer most commonly occurs. Usually the examination is negative, with a complaint of pain localization to one side or other, and when the head of the epididymis organ is squeezed, it reproduces the pain for the patient. Rarely does a vasectomy result in such tenderness or chronic orchalgia.

It is important to understand the nerve supply to the testis so that the diagnostic evaluation can make some functional sense. The pelvic nerve plexus supplies the input, and pain can arise from both the normal sensory nerves and the autonomic nerves. These fibers are carried in the branches of the genitofemoral and ilioinguinal nerves. Findings of fluid around the testicle, varicose veins, or sperm cysts (spermatocele), are usually coincidental and are never the cause of the chronic orchalgia. This pain is almost always epididymal nerve pain and not testicular pain.

Removal of the epididymis as an approach to treat chronic testes pain has met with failure. Slightly more successful when all else has failed has been cutting the nerves, using a microscopic method, to remove all nerve fibers from the spermatic cord arising from the testicular tissue or the scrotal contents. We always perform a selective anesthetic spermatic cord nerve block as a diagnostic and sometimes therapeutic procedure first, adding a cortisone solution to a long-acting anesthetic. Several of these nerve blocks at intervals can sometimes relieve the cyclic nature of this syndrome. A recent report by Dr. Magdy Hassouna from Canada proposes that sacral nerve root electrical stimulation may be beneficial in these patients, and in some cases, skin surface electrical stimulation has been helpful.

Interstitial cystitis: symptoms and treatment

Interstitial cystitis (IC) usually means pelvic pain associated with urinary urgency and frequency. The old diagnosis of urethral syndrome composed of urinary urgency, frequency, dysuria, suprapubic or low back pain, and voiding difficulties, probably should be included as part of the IC syndrome. Dr. Niall Galloway from Emory University proposed that IC represents a type of reflex sympathetic dystrophy of the bladder—too much nerve tone stimulating the muscles and blood vessels. The early symptoms of sympathetic dystrophy include a burning pain and hypersensitivity, the same bladder complaints from IC patients. There may be a spasm of blood vessels feeding the bladder which creates a loss of oxygen to the organ. This phenomenon in other parts of the body causes capillary blood vessel fragility. We note the same blood vessel fragility when stretching the bladder under anesthesia. The vessels rupture, creating small hemorrhages and formation of a characteristic bloody pattern to the surface of the bladder. We describe this as a possible objective criterion to accompany the clinical diagnosis of IC. Occasionally, the stretching procedure done under anesthesia benefits as many as 30% of patients who note sustained improvement in their symptoms. Therefore bladder distention has become a therapeutic tool to manage this condition. Bladder biopsy is rarely necessary, as no significant microscopic findings contribute to management, and no serious diseases are uncovered. If there is anything suspicious, however, superficial bladder cancer needs to be ruled out.

One common concept of IC centers on a defect in the bladder surface mucosal barrier known as the glycosaminoglycan (GAG) layer. Abnormalities in this layer may allow micropores or tiny holes to develop, ultimately allowing urinary metabolites or toxins, especially potassium molecules to invade through the lining to the submucosal receptors of nerves and blood vessels. When a physician introduces potassium solutions into the bladder of someone suffering from IC, the pain induced confirms a susceptibility of "leakage" of noxious stimuli into the submucosa.

There is only one oral drug officially approved by the U.S. Food and Drug Administration for the treatment of IC in an attempt to improve the GAG layer in the bladder. The drug is pentosan polysulfate sodium (Elmiron®). In multiple clinical trials of this drug, 28-40% of all patients have significant improvement after using it. It takes several weeks of therapy, usually from three to six months to reach the greatest benefit. In a recent NIH clinical trial comparing Elmiron® and antihistamine (hydroxyzine), 34% of the patients obtained a response with Elmiron and 18% of the patients obtained a response when taking a sugar pill (placebo). With the antihistamine, 31% of patients obtained a response and 20% taking a sugar pill obtained a response. When both drugs were taken, 40% obtained a response.

Sometimes we instill medications directly into the bladder. Dimethylsulfoxide (DMSO) has been approved for this purpose and reports have indicated that up to 70% of patients experiencing symptomatic remission. Many times the physician will create a "cocktail" with DMSO adding hydrocortisone, alkalinizing sodium bicarbonate, Lidocaine® or Marcaine® (topical anesthetic) and heparin to act as a surface sealant.

Current clinical research is testing immunotherapy with tuberculosis vaccine (BCG) as a treatment for IC. Trials currently underway in the United States hope to reveal the benefits of this agent. Preliminary trials suggest that 65% of these patients using immunotherapy show improvements of their symptoms. Hyalouronic acid (Cyotostat®) has not been approved in the United States, but reports of benefit after placement in the bladder come from Canada.

Surgical treatment of IC uniformly proves unsuccessful, but fortunately less than 5% of patients require surgical treatment. Surgery may include removal of the bladder and urethra and creation of a substitution bladder or pouch from intestine. Sometimes the easiest management is to divert urine with an intestinal conduit to the skin and a urinary collection bag worn on the abdomen. Occasionally, surgical enlargement of the bladder using components of intestine helps. This is particularly true when the bladder has shrunken from chronic inflammation.

Interstitial cystitis appears to afflict primarily young to middle aged women in a ratio of 8 to 1 (female to male). Most women mistakenly carry a diagnosis of urinary tract infection, as in chronic prostatitis with men, and are given a myriad of antimicrobial agents. The cause of IC is completely unknown, but has no cancer-related effects and no documentation of infection. Many investigators have tried to uncover an autoimmunity phenomenon in this disorder.

There has always been a question about the effects of hormones in the woman who is suffering from chronic pelvic pain and IC. In a recent report by Dr. G. M. Lentz from the University of Washington in Seattle, patients who do not have evidence of endometriosis on laparoscopy seem to improve with inhibition of hormonal activity. The patients were treated with oral contraceptive pills and had a high percentage of remission of their symptoms.

One of the confounding issues in chronic pelvic pain syndrome in males is whether the prostate, the bladder, or both are involved. In 1995 researchers at the University of Washington reported that 50% of 20 patients referred for chronic prostatitis had irritated voiding symptoms. Twelve of the 20 patients had the characteristic findings of petechial hemorrhages (pinpoint bleeding) involving the bladder lining when stretched or hydrodistended under anesthesia; there were no other histopathological abnormalities on biopsy.

We commonly fail to diagnose IC in men. These men wander from doctor to doctor with a diagnosis of "chronic prostatitis," when in fact their urinary symptoms suggest possible bladder inflammation more than prostate inflammation. The University of Washington in Seattle claims that as many as 60% of men referred for pelvic pain fit the criteria for diagnosis of IC. These men deserve the benefit of the multimodal medical therapy currently available. It is necessary to be vigilant regarding the complaints of patients with chronic pelvic pain to discover any possible disorders that may respond to treatment even if cure is not possible. *On the other hand, we should not plant suggestions in the mind of the suffering patient that there exists a specific undiscovered organic disorder to explain the condition.*

Hypotheses to explain interstitial cystitis

Similar to sympathetic dystrophy in the hands and feet, bladder IC may arise from a triggering event. A patient may have had urinary infection, surgery, childbirth, some viral illness, or even physical or psychological trauma. Sensations of bladder pain become a focal prominent feature. As in other bodily tissues afflicted by nerve spasticity to arterial blood vessels, the tissues end up developing fibrosis or scarring. This occurs in the bladder of classic IC patients after many years of chronic inflammation. New laboratory research also shows an abnormal protein in the urine of IC patients, which inhibits healthy regeneration of bladder surface cells. There is considerable gathering evidence as espoused by Dr. Tony Buffington, that an imbalance between the cortisone producing endocrine system and hyperactivated nervous system is responsible for the disorder and furthermore, this may have been imprinted with behavioral and genetic predisposition in infancy. Considerably more research is required to sort out the complexities involved here.

The neurovascular insult hypothesis to explain IC suggests the features are secondary to an ongoing bladder damaging process. Drs. Erwin and Galloway treated a large number of patients with painful bladder disorders using nerve blockage at the lumbar level to obliterate the natural adrenaline producing nerve activity in the bladder. This successfully improved immediate pain in a large portion of the patients.

This type of clinical experimental work helps forward our knowledge about the cause of the bladder pain syndrome. The problem may be a neurovascular deficit supplying the bladder with circulating oxygen.

Regardless of causation of this condition, pelvic floor muscle management, particularly of myofascial trigger points, benefits this *group of patients.* Dr. Jerome M. Weiss, a urologist in San Francisco, published a paper reporting his success in treating both men and women with urgency/frequency syndrome, reducing their symptoms with intrapelvic myofascial release treatment. Of the 42 patients with the urgency/ frequency syndrome (with or without pain) for 6 to 14 years, 83% had moderate to marked improvement or complete resolution. He postulates that the bladder is not completely responsible for the symptoms or the urgency/frequency syndrome; the pelvic floor and the sphincter muscles play a major part. These patients typically have tender spots in the pelvis on palpation and it is consistent with the myofascial trigger points we have described. Many patients with the diagnosis of IC describe difficult voiding in childhood and may have had previous trauma contributing to their dysfunction, even triggering events that appear so trivial as to not be recognized as a cause.

Anatomically the pelvic floor myofascial trigger points influence the bladder because their nerve nuclei or origins lie in close proximity within the spinal cord to incoming nerve endings from bladder autonomic nerves. Flare-ups of IC, including pain and urinary urgency, can be activated by stress, dietary indiscretions, improper exercise or movement, trauma, sexual activity, cold weather, hormonal shifts, and viral infection. Dr. Weiss has done a good job at postulating the relationship between the organ bladder dysfunction and discomfort in relationship to the pelvic floor. Details of the actual neurophysiologic changes within the nervous system and within the muscular tissue have yet to be worked out by the basic scientists, but clinicians continue to seek the relationships that may guide basic investigation.

Depressive symptoms and quality of life of patients with interstitial cystitis

A recent publication from the University of Iowa by Dr. Nan Rothrock indicates that a diagnosis of IC relates to poor functioning in various life domains, as obviously the severity of the disease dictates how much the quality of life deteriorates. It is always difficult for the physician, friends and neighbors, and others to appreciate how much disability a chronic pain disorder may have. IC adversely affects leisure activities, family relations, and travel in 70-94% of patients. Depression and fatigue is another common experience of these patients; difficulty concentrating and insomnia are aspects of that as well. It has been stated that patients with IC are 3-4 times more likely to report suicidal thoughts. The University of Iowa study was confined to female patients. In addition to the clinical psychiatric and psychological inventories, microscopic tissue was examined from bladder biopsies. Forty, age-matched, healthy control patients were also asked to complete questionnaires about their depressive symptoms. As expected, those patients with more severe disease had significantly greater limitations in their physical and social functioning as well as mental health. It was interesting to note that in the biopsies of the bladder, inflammation of the bladder was relatively uncommon, and was either not present or mild in 80% of the patients, and ulceration was absent in 80% of the patients. However, 80% of the patients did show moderate to severe capillary fragility with petechial hemorrhages. No specific IC symptom seemed to be primarily associated with depression. The positive note in this study is that although patients had greater depressive symptomatology than healthy control patients, there was very little severe depression and patients were able to cope with normal life experiences.

We continue to question the role of *infections causing IC,* and thus far the quest has come up empty-handed. Dr. Keay at the University of Maryland found a toxic factor in the urine 95% of the time in those patients who had a diagnosis of IC. This factor is a protein that inhibits the normal proliferation or growth of the surface cells in the bladder. Much further investigative work needs to be done to put this into perspective.

One of the common diagnostic tests for IC consists of putting a potassium solution in the bladder and determining whether it causes more pain than simply water. One of the questions about this is whether there is any correlation between the sensitivity of the bladder to this potassium and the finding of the blood vessel fragility on stretching of the bladder. A recent study by Dr. Gergeoire from Quebec, Canada, showed no difference in blood vessel fragility in those who had positive potassium tests and those who did not.

Vulvodynia

Vulvodynia, or hypersensitivity of the vulva and vaginal opening, was described in the 19th century. It includes disorders named *vulvar vestibulitis* and *essential vulvodynia*. The incidence and prevalence of these problems is really not known. Usually 50% of these patients experience dyspareunia or painful sexual intercourse. They feel pain upon penile insertion into the vaginal opening, as well as pain inserting tampons. *Vulvar vestibulitis* means there is a dermatological inflammation at the vaginal entrance with a pronounced redness when touched even lightly. Sharp pain occurs when this delicate skin is rubbed, and this pain prohibits normal sexual intercourse.

Unfortunately this disorder commonly occurs in sexually active young women, and can even develop after normal, non-painful sexual intercourse has occurred before. Occasionally these women will have a coincident occurrence of bladder interstitial cystitis with their vulvodynia disorder. Many women are misdiagnosed as having fungal vaginitis, lichen planus, or contact dermatitis, and are treated with anti-fungal agents and other topical medications; these may even exacerbate or worsen some of the inflammatory responses. Some have suggested a coinciding sub-clinical infection of the human papilloma or genital wart virus, but there is no scientific proof of this relationship.

Patients are typically treated with medications such as antidepressants (Elavil®) for neuropathic pain, topical estrogens, and cortisone creams. *Surgical or destructive manipulations of the tissues have a disappointing outcome.*

CHAPTER 10

HOW TO CONTACT US

We wish our treatment were available everywhere. We get many inquiries from around the world from patients asking how they may undergo this therapy. Unfortunately there are few to whom we can refer at this time.

The person who undergoes this treatment needs a 'quarterback,' someone who sees the overall picture and can guide the patient in therapy through the many ups and downs that inevitably occur.

It is our hope that a groundswell of patients will prompt a reluctant medical community to learn how to treat chronic pelvic pain syndromes using the method discussed in this book. To that end we are designing a program for professionals interested in learning our work.

We offer a monthly 6-day intensive program for out-of-town patients in California using the protocol described in this book. We can be reached in the following ways:

Email: ahip@sonic.net

Telephone: (707) 874-2225
Toll free: (866) 874-2225

Website: www.pelvicpainhelp.com

Mail: National Center for Pelvic Pain
P.O. Box 54
Occidental, CA 95465

Disclaimer

Many readers have found that reading this book has helped them better deal with or reduce their symptoms. This book however is not intended as a self-help book and is not meant to be a substitute for competent medical or psychological diagnosis or treatment. The aim of the Stanford Protocol is to help patients become independent and to be able to reduce or resolve their symptoms themselves without reliance on others. This independence requires training with and consultation by those practitioners whom we have trained in *Paradoxical Relaxation* and *Myofascial/Trigger Point Release*. Our approach is used when medical evaluation has ruled out physical illness and pathology.